COLLEGE OF MARIN LIBRARY
KENTFIELD, CALIFORNIA

SO-BKT-295

MALNOURISHED CHILDREN
OF THE RURAL POOR

MALNOURISHED CHILDREN OF THE RURAL POOR

The Web of Food, Health, Education, Fertility, and Agricultural Production

JUDITH B. BALDERSTON
ALAN B. WILSON
MARIA E. FREIRE
MARI S. SIMONEN
of the Berkeley Project on Education and Nutrition

with Forewords by
CHARLES S. BENSON
SHELDON MARGEN

HV
747
, G9
M34

 Auburn House Publishing Company
Boston, Massachusetts

Copyright © 1981 by Auburn House Publishing Company

All rights reserved. No part of this publication may be reproduced,
translated, or transmitted in any form or by any means without
permission in writing from Auburn House Publishing Company at
131 Clarendon Street, Boston, Massachusetts 02116.

Library of Congress Cataloging in Publication Data
Main entry under title:

Malnourished children of the rural poor.

   Includes bibliographical references and index.   1.   Rural children—
Guatemala—Longitudinal studies.   2.   Rural poor—Guatemala—
Longitudinal studies.   3.   Fertility, Human—Guatemala—Longitu-
dinal studies.   4.   Education—Guatemala—Longitudinal
studies.   5.   Malnutrition—Guatemala—Longitudinal
studies.   6.   Agricultural productivity—Guatemala—
Longitudinal studies.   I.   Balderston, Judith B.
HV747.G9M34   362.7′95′097281   81-3483
ISBN 0-86569-071-5   AACR2

Printed in the United States of America

FOREWORD

by Charles S. Benson

In 1964 James B. Conant wrote, "All over the world today national governments are considering educational problems in revolutionary terms." So it seemed to be. Theodore Schultz, Edward Denison, and other economists had made the case that expansion of schooling leads to economic growth and to the elimination of poverty—which is not quite the same thing. Human capital theory became accepted in the body of neoclassical economics. The greatest impact of the Schultz-Denison argument in the real world occurred not in American or in the rest of Western society, but in the developing nations. Spurred by offers of grants and loans from the World Bank, the Agency for International Development (AID), and other international agencies, Third World countries poured huge sums of money into their education budgets.

I was among the educational planners sent abroad to work in developing countries during the 1960s and I came not to like what I saw happening. True, certain forms of technical education appeared to make a contribution to the economic growth of the country, but these activities were most generally a small part of the total education enterprise. What seemed patently false was the idea that educational expansion, pursued as a single major isolated policy initiative, did much to help poor people. In the first place, children of poor people do not attend school very long. Even when a poverty child manages to make it through the grades, he (she) tends to do rather badly in examinations. In the second place, educational expansion usually is associated with a rise in credentialism of the monetarized sector of the job market, so less-educated groups in the population get themselves more securely locked out of economic opportunity than they ever were before. Reflecting on my experiences in 1970, I wrote the following:

> *An adviser in education feels conscience-bound to join with those in government, and outside, who argue for raising the amounts of global allocations to education. He may also feel it necessary to plead for*

v

increased allocations to those kinds of services that seem to offer benefits to the masses, rather than those that serve, for the most part, the elite. In my experience, the adviser and his local colleagues are likely to be more successful in the former venture than the latter, rhetoric of plan documents notwithstanding. So no matter what his intentions, the (education) adviser becomes a handmaiden of the entrenched ruling classes. Education is not dealt with in revolutionary terms, contrary to Conant.

The radical economist might say that no one should expect education or expansion of an educational system to bring about a change in the class structure because the educational system exists to assure social reproduction. But the needs of social reproduction do not demand that the poor people of developing nations be as desperately poor as they now are. Consequently, it occurred to me that perhaps social policies for human development are too narrowly defined. In the case of education, for example, we hear a lot about "quality of teacher," meaning the teacher's competence to instruct, but seldom anything significant about the quality of student, meaning the student's physical and mental competence to learn. Let's put it in terms of a trade-off of resources. As seen by a village, educational expansion means adding another room to the schoolhouse and hiring another teacher. If our goal is social mobility, it might be better to spend the extra resources, or some of them, in another way, namely, to improve the health of low-income children, so that they may enter school more readily, and, once there, pay attention.

It was from raising such questions that I had a modest share in helping the project get started. The outcome far exceeds my early hopes. The authors are able for the first time to examine thoroughly the effects on very young children of several social interventions pursued simultaneously—among them, nutrition, health, and education—and to conduct this examination with the benefit of detailed knowledge of the context of family and village.

A note of caution. In the chapter on policy conclusions it is suggested that the goal of social mobility requires a concentrated effort along several difficult lines all at once. If poor people are to benefit, we need to be concerned simultaneously about nutrition, health, education, family planning, cooperative work arrangements, and so on. The reader may be inclined to throw up his (her) hands and say, "But if it will all cost so much money, it's impossible." It will cost great effort and persistence in planning, true, but actually not too much money, not necessarily in the setting of the developing world.

Much of what is proposed could be done rather cheaply, especially if local professionals were prepared to perform more than one set of tasks. The main difficulty to be overcome in establishing a more complete, integrated, and therefore effective program to help poor children reach their human potential is the fragmented, and often competitive, structure of social service agencies in Third World countries. It is a problem known to us in the United States as well.

FOREWORD

by Sheldon Margen

In the flush of exuberance at the end of World War II, just as we finally felt free of the scourge of war, pestilence, and poverty, the now-deceased Lloyd Boyd Orr struck a note of alarm: He told us that two thirds of the world's children went to bed starving and malnourished every night! However, in the euphoria of the immediate postwar period, many interpreted this not as a warning, but as a challenge. The world was at the threshold of change and all would share in the benefits, if not equally, at least to a greater degree. But alas, now more than forty years later, the problems are still with us, not only in absolute numbers, but also in greater magnitude.

As the solutions continue to elude us, and poverty and inequity continue to mount, we have seen that, of all the effects, the associations with malnutrition appear to be the most pernicious. To a great extent high infant mortality in developing countries can be attributed either to malnutrition per se or to complications that occur in weakened, nutritionally deprived children.

Poverty and food deprivation move hand in hand; not all the poor are malnourished, but virtually all the malnourished are poor. As world leaders grow to understand that poverty and hunger are not about to disappear, new questions arise. What causes malnutrition and poverty? These conditions were found to be embedded in such a complex morass of sociocultural, economic, and political factors that short-range solutions were totally impossible. Somehow we are becoming inured to the spectre of death. The dead cannot cry out for justice. They cannot revolt. What of those who have been malnourished and manage to survive? What is their future? What kind of life may the ill-fed expect to live? What kind of permanent impairments will they suffer? How many of the malnourished exist? Are their physical and mental impairments so great that they cannot escape the web of poverty and deprivation? Are they incapable of learning or competing both as individuals and as societies because of irrevocable injuries suffered from malnutrition and illness in childhood? Would special food programs for pregnant mothers and children alleviate this? These are important questions but they are asked in a spirit of humanity, not understanding.

Before the questions and problems have been carefully analyzed, however, policies have been instituted to alleviate "the situation." Massive feeding programs, development of high-protein foods, and a concentration on calories have all been proposed as the *solution*. But the *problem* has yet to be clearly defined. Extensive studies were set up to determine the effects of mild-to-moderate food deprivation on "mental development." Not only was the definition and measurement of mental process difficult; it became clear that all types of social deprivations—including food—could lead to serious deficits of mental development. The waters became increasingly muddy. But our group in Berkeley, studying education and nutrition, decided to plunge in anyway. We had no illusions that we would come up with "answers," definitions of the problems, or suggestions of specific policy. By and large, we got into this "because it was there," and we wanted to see what we might learn.

We examined one broad, complex, major experiment and found many startling conclusions. The findings speak clearly for themselves, but a certain murkiness must prevail because, as with all research, the presence and past of experimenter and analyst become part of the results. The interpretations of our findings will also be modified by the reader. For our part, if this book can contribute to saving one child from death, deprivation, illness, or hunger, we would all feel our work was not in vain.

PREFACE

It is hard to avoid statistics about poverty, hunger, infant mortality, and widespread malnutrition. Almost every day the grim facts are placed before us—sometimes in appeals for charitable contributions, but more often in discussions of the interdependencies of world economics and politics.

For many years the majority view among development economists was that poverty and malnutrition could be alleviated by economic development. The World Bank, which typified this view, shifted its position in 1980 to call attention to the basic needs of those continuing to live in absolute poverty. In its latest *World Development Report* (1980, p. 32) the Bank comments:

> The case for human development is not only, or even primarily an economic one. Less hunger, fewer child deaths, and a better chance of primary education are almost universally accepted as important ends in themselves. But in a world of tight budgetary and manpower constraints, the governments of developing countries must ask what these gains would cost, and what the best balance is between direct and indirect ways of achieving them.

No matter how gains are measured—in terms of economic growth, of alleviating absolute poverty, or of distributing income more equitably—the improvement of living conditions for the poor will continue to be of central importance for international aid agencies and governments. The analytical study upon which this book is based was undertaken by the Berkeley Project on Education and Nutrition in order to contribute to understanding more fully the consequences of poverty, particularly poor health, malnutrition, and illiteracy. We hoped that, by looking at interrelationships among these conditions, we would be able to offer some directions for remedial policies.

When we began, we expected to see a set of well-researched and measured interrelationships; we were surprised, however, to find that many unexplored areas existed. We had to retreat from our intended approach as policy analysts and begin our work in the research domain. In conducting this research we found also that we could not limit ourselves to the original areas of interest but had to enlarge the study to include other dimensions of life, such as the determinants of family size and farm productivity. We were able to examine many aspects of lives of people in rural communities in Guatemala and, at the completion of our analysis, to combine separate conclusions into a more comprehensive whole.

We began with the search for relationships between nutrition and education and the out-of-school performance of young people. Originally the study was undertaken to (1) test hypotheses regarding the relationships between education, health, and nutrition, particularly with respect to the effect of nutrition on school performance and activities of children; and (2) analyze how acceptance of nutritional supplementation, health care, contraception, and education relate to family income, parental literacy, and education. At the time the study was proposed and funded it was suggested that our work would "be useful in predicting the effects of early malnutrition on later stages in the life cycle and how early growth and development are related to success in school and in the performance of economic activities."

To carry out such an investigation requires collecting data in a wide variety of areas—physiological, nutritional, socioeconomic, psychological—and in a natural-setting environment where the interaction among areas would take place and be observed. It was therefore extremely fortunate that the ambitious and costly longitudinal study by INCAP (*Institute of Nutrition of Central America and Panama*)—funded by the National Institute of Child Health and Development between 1969 and 1978, and by RAND (through Rockefeller Foundation funding), in 1974–1975—had already taken place in the four villages in Eastern Guatemala. Because a large and varied data base had been amassed out of these projects it was possible to make the connections between children's individual growth and development, their families' economic and social conditions, and the environment of the village economies and schools. It was hoped that results (obtained through the use of appropriate analytical models) would be useful for policy formulation in international agencies, mainly by stressing the importance of intersectoral planning in less-developed countries.

At the time of our proposal it was recognized that, although much was already known about effects of severe malnutrition, the result of chronic malnutrition on human functioning deserved much more investigation. Nutritional science, well developed in the laboratory, had not yet been able to translate known chemical and biological relationships into functional outcomes. The purpose of INCAP's ambitious study had been to see how some nutritional and health inputs related to growth and development outcomes. The Berkeley study aimed to enable educational and other planners to see how nutritional change might affect educational outcomes.

To integrate plans made separately by organizations in various fields—such as nutrition, public health, rural development, and education—would potentially improve the cost-effectiveness of programs. Since such integration requires knowledge of relationships between separate sectors, it was suggested that data from the INCAP and RAND studies in Guatemala would provide many important research results.

The chapters of this book represent the work carried out by the members of the Berkeley Project. Chapter 1 discusses the need for research, Chapter 2, the background of the Guatemalan study. Chapters 3 through 6 present the analytical studies, using the Guatemalan data: Chapter 3, longitudinal analysis of diet, growth, development, and school performance; Chapter 4, determinants of school participation; Chapter 5, the relationship of schooling to agricultural efficiency; Chapter 6, the relationship of schooling to fertility. In Chapter 7 we discuss the policy implications of the research findings.

We hope these findings will be of interest and importance to those responsible for making plans in a variety of sectors. The data base is so rich that we have only been able to tap a small part of it. We expect, and hope, that others will go further by using the information from INCAP and RAND as well as undertaking related studies in other places. It is unlikely that such an ambitious collection of data will be made again; instead, lessons learned from the strengths and weaknesses of the INCAP and Berkeley efforts will assist researchers who follow. We believe that some results of our investigation could indicate definite policy steps, while others will need to be further clarified.

We are grateful for the financial support of the United States Agency for International Development. Our research results and discussions of policy implications are, however, our own and not those of AID.

Professors Charles Benson and Sheldon Margen undertook to

oversee the Berkeley Project on Education and Nutrition as Co-Principal Investigators. Judith Balderston was Project Director and Alan Wilson, Maria Freire, and Mari Simonen were involved throughout the project. Although this work represented a group effort, individuals took responsibility for separate parts of the analysis. The names of the separate authors identify the individual chapters of the book.

We are grateful indeed to INCAP, the National Institute for Child Health and Development, and the National Science Foundation who supported the tremendous data collection in Guatemala. Many people associated with INCAP were very helpful to us: Robert Klein who directed the study, William Owens, Charles Yarbrough, Marc Irwin, John Townsend, and Reynaldo Martorell. We are also grateful for the support of the Rockefeller Foundation in the extremely valuable RAND study. Dr. William Butz at RAND was especially generous in providing data and taking time to help us. Patricia Engle and Carol Clark both were helpful and knowledgeable sources of information on RAND and INCAP data.

We thank the staff at AID, particularly Dr. Anthony Meyer, and the members of the research review committee, Drs. Sam Wishik, Laurence Lau, and Henry Ricciuti, whose comments were of great benefit in interpreting our results.

Several members of the Berkeley staff do not appear as authors but participated, nevertheless, in crucial activities. Jane Fraser's massive organization of the data base was essential to our work. Vien Phan and Patsy Fosler prepared files for analysis. Jo-Ann Work shared much of the administrative burden. Lynne Reilly energetically kept up with the paper flow of so many authors. Marie-Anne Seabury helped us translate our technical language into English. Helen Green made it possible to finish the book on time. We thank them all. The ultimate responsibility is with those of us whose names are found on the individual chapters.

J.B.B.

CONTENTS

LIST OF TABLES

LIST OF FIGURES

Chapter 1

INVESTIGATING THE WEB OF POVERTY—THE NEED FOR RESEARCH

by Judith B. Balderston

> *. . . poverty in modern nations is not only a state of economic deprivation or disorganization or of the absence of something. It is also something positive in the sense that it has a structure, a rationale, and defense mechanisms without which the poor could hardly carry on. In short it is a way of life, remarkably stable and persistent, passed down from generation to generation along family lines. The culture of poverty has its own modalities and distinctive social and psychological consequences for its members. It is a dynamic factor which affects participation in the larger national culture and becomes a subculture of its own.*
>
> Oscar Lewis, *The Children of Sanchez* (Random House, 1961)

> *. . . poor children are not merely born* into *poverty; they are born* of *poverty. . . .*
>
> Herbert Birch and Joan Gussow, *Disadvantaged Children: Health, Nutrition and School Failure* (Harcourt Brace and World, Inc., 1970)

> *It is difficult to measure the extent of poverty. To begin with, absolute poverty means more than low income. It also means malnutrition, poor health, and lack of education . . . .*
>
> The World Bank, *World Development Report*, 1980

1

Children of poor rural families are caught in an intergenerational web of multiple hazards: malnutrition, poor health, illiteracy, poor housing, and lack of economic and social opportunity. To extricate them from a web so stable, persistent, and damaging calls for major and difficult change. Because of the great number of poor people and the ubiquity of poverty, even comparatively minor changes in individual lives become huge overall investments. And it may be especially hard to justify investing even in such basic needs as public health, nutrition, and education if enhanced economic productivity and development, or more equitable distribution of income, cannot be demonstrated.

The effects of poverty and failure are all too evident in many parts of the world. At birth and during the earliest months of life many children face health hazards that have long-term effects on growth and development. In addition, continuing nutritional deprivation and ill-health tend to cause ongoing and increasing damage, which become handicaps to work and learning.

The child in the impoverished family and community thus is multiply deprived. Because of poverty, the child typically is malnourished and in poor health, the effects of diet and health interacting and magnifying. Growth is stunted due to poor prenatal and early diet. Health conditions of the family are miserable because of overcrowded, makeshift housing without potable water and sanitation. Adult family members, also having known poverty and deprivation, are likely to be poorly nourished, and to suffer from disease; also, typically illiterate, they work at low levels of productivity and for very low pay. Under such inauspicious conditions the child begins life with few opportunities.

Already limited by the physical and developmental consequences of this environment, children are further restricted by the economic need for them to work which begins at a very early age. Parents who feel that the (very pressing) need for children's present work outweighs future (remote) benefits in increased earnings are unlikely to let their children go to school. And the absence of education, which acts as an agent for economic opportunity, may further handicap the child's future.

The malnourished child living in rural poverty faces a bleak future, similar to the parents' past. From generation to generation, in fact, these conditions may be worsened by increased population and depleted natural resources. Such mutually reinforcing deprivations increase the deficits; poor diet and health affect the physical capacity of children to explore and interact with the environment.

Therefore, it is not surprising that physical damage is done to the developing child and that economic and intellectual potentials are curtailed. It *is* surprising that the human body is adaptable enough to survive and to cope with severe physical and psychological stress. Despite high mortality and morbidity rates, individuals and families *do* survive, using modes of coping developed over generations. Biological adaptation means that the child's body grows more slowly—beginning with lower birth-weight, maturing later than the nondeprived, attaining shorter stature, and leading to more restricted physical activity than would result from an adequate diet. Economic patterns are similarly adaptive: Risk is avoided whenever possible; the labor of all family members is used; family size (large) reflects high infant mortality and the need for children's work. Since extended families often live together, these social patterns persist across generations. The child who has suffered all these deprivations therefore needs several kinds of assistance simultaneously.

We must emphasize here that we shall be looking at poverty through the individual and the family—in technical terms, at the microlevel. The solutions we suggest also will be focused on the individual. We shall not take up questions of the aggregate effects of microchanges, nor shall we address sweeping changes, such as land reform. Our work has been limited to examining the network of relationships that affect individuals; other researchers and policy analysts will be able to use our results for macropolicy analysis.

Moreover, we shall concentrate on the *rural* family. Farm families are different from urban families; because the children can contribute to family income by participating in farm production, there are alternatives to school attendance. Also, for members of farm families, diet depends on the efficiency, productivity, and knowledge of the farmer, and these may depend in turn on his prior health, nutrition, and education. Therefore, interdependencies among food, health, schooling, and productivity are especially strong for rural populations.

It is necessary to know if characteristics of poverty are related or are, rather, separate and distinct consequences of low income. When poverty is viewed statistically, it is apparent that malnutrition, disease, illiteracy, low income, low productivity, and large family size are highly correlated. We suspect that one condition tends to exacerbate another: Poor health makes malnutrition worse; illiteracy produces low economic opportunity; high infant mortality leads to the need for larger families; poor health causes school absenteeism and failure. Some of these relationships may be physiological in nature; others may result from the interaction of traditional economic and cultural patterns with physiological conditions. In order to intervene successfully and efficiently, it is important to disentangle these relationships.

Need for Research

Social programs for development have tended to emphasize education, educational planning, and educational expansion. These programs have assumed that by increasing literacy and skills needed for work, individuals and communities would realize increased productivity, higher income, and, eventually, higher levels of consumption. But educational expansion alone has not been able to solve the problem of abject poverty. In fact, education appears to serve best those students who have not suffered early deprivation. Students who profit most from education come from families of relatively higher income and social class, while children who do not enroll at all—or who fail, repeat, or drop out—most often come from families at the lowest income levels. Thus the promise that schooling will raise individuals out of poverty often is empty.

For developing countries such indications are consistent and clear. A number of studies show that parental income, wealth, social class, and race are strong predictors of children's school achievement (see, for example, Alexander and Simmons, 1975; Sharma and Sapra, 1969). Direct causes of these strong statistical relationships are not always so clear. In fact, the most critical determinants of school success or failure may be factors overlooked in these investigations—early diet, health, physical growth, and cognitive development.

A few recent research efforts have undertaken to examine explicitly the relationships between early childhood nutrition, health, and school performance. In these (see, for example, Weinberg et al., 1974), data analyzed by multiple regression techniques provide estimates of the effect of height or head circumference (as measures of prior nutrition and health) in predicting educational outcomes. Bigger children consistently do better in school, remain in school longer, and show higher test scores.

Proper interpretation of these results requires more thorough knowledge of physiological and developmental processes—how diet and health affect physical size and cognitive growth; how diet, health, and their outcomes are affected by the environment. A great deal of important research (especially in the nutritional and health sciences) has gone into delineating methods of analysis. Regrettably, less attention has been paid to investigating the functional effects of health and nutrition. The absence of such research was noted by the National Research Council in its report, *World Food and Nutrition Study, The Potential Contributions of Research* (National Academy of Sciences, 1977, p. 65):

> *For the individual and for society, there is a need to determine the consequences of low levels of nutrition on work performance, frequency and severity of infection, physical and mental growth and development, school and job performance, pregnancy and lactation, and fertility and family planning. Research should emphasize how diets affect childbearing and childrearing functions. Information is needed on the extent to which the nutritional status of mothers affects the three variables that determine the biological potential for population growth: span of reproductive years, pace at which successive pregnancies occur, and rate of child survival. To decide which nutritional problems should receive priority and how resources may best be allocated among various target groups, it is essential to know the relative seriousness of different states of nutrition and the degree of benefit that can be derived from specific increments of nutritional improvement.*

Research in the nutritional and health sciences has involved hundreds of experiments, countless research papers. This abundance of research activity makes it difficult for social scientists and planners to find out what has been done and what is known. In order to build on some of these findings, we shall sketch very briefly the methods and findings of work undertaken by biological and nutritional scientists. Following that, we shall also indicate a few related areas of work in the social sciences.

Three types of studies have been conducted on malnutrition and its effects: deprivation studies, retrospective studies, and prospective longitudinal studies. Animal experiments, chiefly with rodents and primates, have looked at the effect of food and stimulus deprivation on brain development, birth-weight, and later behavior. The advantage of using animals as models for human development is obvious, since several generations occur in a short time period, and brain structure can be examined in autopsy. The disadvantage is clear also, since species develop at different rates, with distinct gestational and maturational stages. Thus, depending on the species chosen, periods of prenatal malnutrition may have quite different effects on the developing animal. Despite these drawbacks, animal experiments have been helpful for understanding biological structure.

Human deprivation studies have established how children who have suffered early episodes of severe malnutrition compare to control groups at a later date. A problem in assessing these studies is that the early trauma and hospitalization may have had a greater effect than the malnutrition itself.

Retrospective studies, using historical data, have analyzed the effects of socioeconomic status, health, and nutritional factors on a number of behavioral outcomes, including school performance. These studies are sometimes called "ecological" because they view populations in the natural state without introducing interventions exogenously. In one such study (Christiansen *et al.*, 1974), the problem of over- or under-estimation of nutritional effects on performance is made explicit; such difficulties in estimation occur because of the potentially complex relationship between nutrition and a variety of attitudinal social and environmental variables.

Prospective studies, in which interventions will be introduced in a quasi-experimental way, may offer the best methods available for observing the relation of nutritional and other interventions to behavioral effects. Because food deprivation experiments with human subjects are not ethically permissible, quasi-experiments—which introduce beneficial interventions in the natural setting—have been used to test for differences in outcomes between experimental and control groups. Commonly, longitudinal records are kept on relatively small homogeneous populations or on larger, more heterogeneous groups. The major problem in intervention programs, where participation is voluntary, is the possibility of confounding due to self-selection.

Using these three basic methods of data collection, results have been amassed in the following areas: nutrition and health relationships; effects of nutrition and health on physical growth; effects of nutrition and health on neurological structure; and relationships between nutrition, health, growth, cognitive development, and the environment. We shall now turn to a short summary of each of these areas.

Summary of Research Areas

Nutrition and Health

Nutrition and health appear to be closely (almost obviously) related conditions. A healthy organism, unlike an unhealthy one, can use efficiently the nutrients it ingests (see, for example, McFarlane, 1976). Susceptibility to infectious disease appears to be increased when the infant or child has suffered from a combination of malnutrition and infection over a period of time (Rosenberg *et al.*, 1976).

Malnutrition is not just a simple deprivation of food, but a more complicated interaction of nutrient needs and health, based on the level of metabolic and activity processes and the presence of infection. Below a certain level of health or nutrition, the organism simply cannot survive, while accommodation does appear possible within other acceptable ranges. What makes some survive and others go under is not yet sufficiently understood, although research continues. Chen and colleagues (see Chen, Rahman, and Sarder, 1980, and Chen, Huq, and Huffman, 1980) have been working to establish better connections between nutrition and disease in their work on cholera and diarrhea in Bangladesh.

Nutrition, Health, and Growth

Stunting and wasting occur as a result of prenatal malnutrition, the mother's general health and nutritional state, her condition during lactation, and the child's early diet. Not all maternal, prenatal malnutrition appears to affect fetal growth and development similarly, however. Stein and Susser *et al.* (1975), studying the Dutch famine of 1944–1945, showed that when the mother's prior condition is good, an episode of starvation will not affect the baby's birth-weight and subsequent development. It is believed that below a nutritional threshold, however, the fetus is vulnerable and cannot develop normally (see Stein and Susser, 1976). In an earlier study of children born during the siege of Leningrad (1941–1942), Antonov (1947) concluded that the condition of the mother's body is of great importance to the developing fetus.

In spite of a large number of studies of maternal malnutrition and birth-weight, the mechanism by which maternal nutritional intake affects the baby's size at birth is not completely clear. Low-birth-weight babies have been shown to suffer other kinds of retardation (see, for example, Drillien, 1960; Birch, 1972) which may be caused by the same mechanism as low birth-weight, or by limiting an infant's ability to function, explore, and learn.

In experimental animal studies prenatal malnutrition has been shown to affect birth-weight and the subsequent ability of the animal to explore the environment (see, for example, Frankova, 1974). The severity of effects of prenatal malnutrition, as observed in animal experiments, appears to be related to the length of time, and developmental period, of the malnutrition.

Recent work by Tanner (1976, 1978), Seckler (1980), and Chen, Chowdury, and Huffman (1980) challenges the long-held "deprivation theory of growth." That theory assumed a given, genetically determined potential growth curve at birth for every properly nourished, healthy individual. More recently, a "homeostatic theory of growth" postulates a multifactorial, "smart gene" that controls the individual's response to the environment. Tanner suggests that the single, potential growth curve be replaced by a growth space, the bounds of which are set genetically; nutritional and environmental factors shape the exact growth curve traced by the growing child. Under this theory the physiological clock is regulated by the relation between the supply and demand of nutrients, and a series of short-term equilibria will trace a smooth course of growth and development. When bounds are exceeded, however, short-term equilibria are replaced by an unstable path; balance is destroyed, and function may be impaired. Tanner thus may offer a key to the difference between moderate malnourishment—in which functional impairments are not noticeable—and severe malnourishment—in which function breaks down. This theory shows that it is possible for people to be small but healthy and that, within limits, size and function do adjust.

Protein-Calorie Relationships and Growth

During the 1950s and 1960s protein-energy malnutrition (PEM) was believed to be a serious problem, particularly in developing countries. Later, in the 1970s, continuing research led to a decision that protein alone was not the limiting factor (Sukhatme, 1977); instead, low total-caloric intake was what restricted growth and development (Milner, 1976). INCAP's nutritional supplementation experiment in Guatemala began during the earlier period in which protein was considered limiting. The nature of the INCAP experiment was to investigate the relationship between protein and calories (prenatally, and during early childhood) to the child's physical growth and mental development. The INCAP experiment will be discussed at length in later chapters of this book.

Nutrition and Brain Development

Extreme changes in structural brain development and in neurophysiological levels may be produced by undernutrition and hormonal imbalance. Undernutrition during key periods of brain development in laboratory animals or humans results in apparently irreversible deficits in cell number and brain weight (see Dobbing and Smart, 1974; Prescott, Read, and Coursin, 1974).

Many investigations have been undertaken on the topic of malnutrition and development of the nervous system (see Sourander *et al.*, 1974). Dobbing (1976) and Winick (1976) both refer to the phase of greatest brain growth as one of the most vulnerable periods of development. Many studies—using laboratory animals, as well as a few investigating human beings—show that PEM may affect the physical development of the nervous system. The number of brain cells, the weight and chemical composition of the brain, the spinal and peripheral nerves, all are affected by nutritional status at crucial times.

Nutritional Effects on Structure, Growth, and Function of the Nervous System

Animal studies have been particularly helpful in explaining nutritional effects—not only on structure and growth of the central nervous system, but also on its functioning. Many investigators have performed animal experiments in which there was early malnutrition and later rehabilitation (see, for example, Barnes *et al.*, 1968). Apparently, early protein-calorie deprivation creates lasting effects upon behavior, some of which can be altered through later enrichment of diet but which do not completely disappear. Both mild and severe malnutrition appear to affect learning. Some abnormalities appear to be due to stunting, which in turn affects exploratory behavior; as a result of early deprivation, other abnormalities seem related to a much greater interest in food than in other stimuli. This is considered by some to be an adaptation of the organism in order to guarantee survival.

Frankova (1974) suggests that early malnutrition causes behavioral abnormalities in experimental animals. Rats with protein-calorie deprivation appear to show less exploratory activity and fewer interactions both with littermates and the mother. Some of this damage can be repaired by increased stimulation of the infant animal. Frankova (1968) shows that early adverse nutrition can be altered but that effects are relative to the size of litter—later stimulation having less effect in extremely large litters. However, stimulation combined with a high-fat diet appeared to compensate for early malnutrition. In other work, Frankova and Barnes (1968) showed that the timing—whether malnutrition occurred before or after weaning—apparently led to different behavioral results. Levitsky (1975) showed that malnutrition produces decreased interaction between an animal and the environment, delaying the development of behavior that would allow the rat to leave its mother and explore its environment independently. Apparently, malnourished animals avoid novel objects in the environment and exhibit exaggerated reactions to unpleasant stimuli.

Recent work by Rosenzweig and Bennett has indicated that the nervous system is relatively plastic. Change in structure of the nervous system is seen to occur if the environment provides certain kinds of stimuli (Rosenzweig, 1980, and Rosenzweig and Bennett, 1980).

Psychologists believe that there is a strong parallel between animal and human behavior, in that the human infant also, if optimally fed and in good health, is responsive to the environment, reacts to stimuli at an early age, and thereby accumulates experience which is the basis for learning and behavior (see, for example, Ricciuti, 1977). An apathetic child—possibly apathetic because of poor nutrition and health—has little interest in exploring the environment, but stays close to the comforting presence of the mother, thereby minimizing the effect of new stimuli and experience. Since maternal attention may be greater toward the inquisitive and demanding child, the amount of interaction between mother and child therefore will be greater for an active child (Chavez and Martinez, 1979).

Malnutrition, Physiology, and Function in the Environment

Retrospective studies have related anthropometric indications of past nutrition and health and social indications of family income and education with cognitive and behavioral outcomes. The intent in such studies is to model how nutrition and health, in the environment, affect function. But, since family nutrition and health may be highly correlated with family education and income, the model that would make relationships explicit is simultaneously important and difficult to construct.

The environment and the nutrition and health of the family interact closely in two ways. First, nutrition and health conditions may result directly from family income and knowledge. Second, the physiological effects of nutrient intake, interacting with the environment, affect the way the child functions in that environment.

The first set of relationships—between nutrition and health, and family wealth and background—can sometimes be controlled by statistical means. In multiple regression analysis it is possible to test for the independent effects of nutrition and health, if data are adequate. Nutritional intervention studies are useful since they allow improvement in family diet independent of family economic status.

The second set of relationships—between nutrition, health, and the environment—makes research more challenging. There may be a cognitive analogy here to the Tanner growth model. Perhaps there is a cognitive growth space, whose upper limit is defined by genetic potential and by early nutrition and health. The mother's own early childhood health and nutrition, her pre-pregnancy condition, and her diet and health during pregnancy affect her infant at birth. Before weaning, the mother's condition continues to affect the infant physically; the manner in which she and the infant respond to each other will have long-range behavioral consequences. At each stage the child's developmental path will result from earlier conditions, the environment, and the nature of experience to that point. The amount of physical vigor—essential to gaining independent experience at each stage—may be limited by the available and usable nutrients. If the nutrient supply exceeds nutrient need (for metabolic, and other processes), then the body will be able to reach the activity level necessary for this exploration. If there is a deficit of nutrients, or if disease prevents their utilization, then activity, and therefore experience, may be curtailed.

Animal experiments have shown this interrelation of the organism with the environment, whether the behavior is inquisitive and exploratory or fearful and clinging. Cognition appears to develop from experience in the environment, and this knowledge and awareness depends on the level of activity, vigor, neural development, and on the environment itself (Frankova, 1974).

Several recent studies have compared exploratory behavior of malnourished children with adequately nourished control groups (see, for example, Graves, 1976). Other studies have looked at later performance of children who have recovered from severe malnourishment in infancy and who are examined at school age (see, for example, Richardson, 1979). A number of similar recent studies are summarized by Pollitt (1979). In all of these studies the model must acknowledge that socioeconomic status (SES) may be highly correlated with nutrition, health, and parental education if it is to be successful in explaining how nutrition affects function.

Early work by Cravioto and DeLicardie (1968) and Monckeberg (1968) emphasized the need for prospective, experimental, longitudinal work. It was recognized that carefully conceived intervention studies would be necessary for collecting adequate data: During the early 1970s the National Institute of Child Health and Development and the Rockefeller Foundation helped to organize and support longitudinal work (Read, 1979). The INCAP experiment was one of these; other studies, financed by the Rockefeller Foundation, followed the effects of nutritional and stimulation interventions.

Due to the necessary expense and time, only a few longitudinal studies have been undertaken. These studies have been carried out in Cali, Colombia by the McKays *et al.* (1978); by Mora *et al.* (1974) in Bogota; by Chavez and Martinez in Mexico (1975); and by Klein and colleagues at INCAP in Guatemala (1977). Brozek (1979) contains papers describing the work of all four groups involved in these studies. Intervention studies are an improvement over correlational studies since, in the latter, nutritional deficiencies may be confounded with the effects of poverty. Moreover, intervention studies make it possible to measure nutritional status independently of body size; frequently nutritional status is measured by body size, but body size may have been affected by genetic as well as environmental factors.

In these intervention studies the effects of carefully measured nutritional interventions are monitored. Two studies (in Mexico and Guatemala) confine their work to nutritional intervention. In the other two (in Colombia) the intervention combines the nutritional with the psychological. These are all quasi-experimental studies in that a variety of environmental variables cannot be controlled; however, the attempt is made to assess, and to account for, noncontrolled variables in the statistical models.

Briefly, these experiments show that there is an association of birth-weight and later performance. Nutritional intervention does appear to increase birth-weight, although the results are not yet completely clear. Behavioral changes, observed in the Guatemalan and Mexican studies, appear to show that nutritional intervention alone may account for bigger and cognitively more advanced children. The nutritional and educational intervention studies show that the longer the treatment period, the greater effect of the treatment; and, the younger the child, the greater the impact of the intervention. These studies leave open some questions concerning the measurement of home diet and its relation to the nutritional intervention—that is, whether the supplement is really supplementary or is a substitute for home diet.

In the chapters that follow we shall use data collected in the Guatemalan study, whose original purpose was to study the functional effects of malnutrition on children in four selected rural communities in Guatemala. INCAP has published a great many papers to date (see, for example, Klein *et al.*, 1974, 1977, 1979) which show that:

1. Birth-weight is determined mainly by the physical characteristics of the mother at the time of conception; height and weight are the most important. Since these are strongly dependent on social class and on the early nutritional status of the mother (when between the ages of one and seven), low birth-weight is likely to repeat for generations, unless specific, counteractive measures are introduced.
2. Birth-weight appears to influence mental development during the first fifteen months of life.
3. Physical growth, as a proxy of child's nutritional status, is seen to depend chiefly on environmental conditions and to be independent of genetic factors.
4. Factors affecting mental development have not yet been determined. There appears to be a relationship between supplementation and test scores.

INCAP's final reports, based on its own analysis of the data, are not yet available. Analysis and interpretation of the INCAP data is expected to be an important and continuing activity for those who want guidance in formulating nutritional policy.

Effects of Literacy and Modernity on Nutrition and Health

Nutrition and health conditions of the family are not totally determined by the environment but can be altered by the decisions made by consumers about what they buy, grow, eat, and how they control sanitation and infection in the household. It may be that healthier children come from families in which the knowledge and attitudes of household decision-makers have created a healthier environment. Sparse research has been done on this topic so far, although there is growing interest in carrying out empirical investigations. Recently, a large empirical analysis for a U.S. population by Coate and Chernichovsky (1980) investigates this issue. The authors find that protein intake significantly affects children's growth, but that family income and education do not determine that nutrient intake. Other related work by Edwards and Grossman (1979), sponsored by the National Bureau of Economic Research, indicates that (in a U.S. white population) family characteristics, especially mother's schooling, do have a significant impact on adolescents' health. These interesting results call for further research, in the context of the developing country.

Nutrition, Health, and School Performance

On the relationship between family characteristics and school achievement, a large literature has developed that shows a strong positive relationship between family socioeconomic status and children's school performance (see, for example, the comprehensive bibliography in Cohn, 1979). What part nutrition and health play in this relationship is unclear and needs to be explored fully. Recent work (see, for example, Popkin and Lim-Ybanez, 1980) has been focused on the relationship of nutrition and health to schooling, in order to improve planning and investing in these areas of social concern.

Nutrition, Health, and Work Productivity

Outcomes of nutrition, health, and education are important for work productivity. Much literature in the field of the economics of education relates the amount of schooling to productivity. Many rate-of-return studies have shown the effect of education on income (see, for example, Psacharopoulos, 1973; a recent summary by Coldough, 1980; and in Cohn, 1979).

The effect of nutrition and health on worker productivity—because of greater physical capacity or mental competence—interests many contemporary investigators (Latham, 1974). Current work at the World Bank by Reutlinger (1980), Selowsky (1978),

Srinvasan (1980), Knudsen and Scandizzo (1979), shows the desire to study these relationships, vis-à-vis policy planning. Interesting theoretical models have been developed by Selowsky (1980). Recent empirical work has shown that more vigorous, well-nourished workers are more productive.

Nutrition, Health, and Fertility

Recent articles have discussed the effects of nutrition and health on fertility (see Butz and Habicht, 1976; Winikoff and Brown, 1980). Close relationships exist among high infant mortality, poor nutrition, and high fertility. If providing better health and nutrition lowers infant mortality, then parents may be more willing to accept contraceptive services. Biological relationships between the mother's nutrition and health and her fecundity, and between breast-feeding and fertility have also been investigated. These areas are especially important for the planning of interventions.

In the following chapters, other areas of research will be described that involve many of the areas discussed above. Reference to other writing will be presented in each of these chapters.

The Berkeley Study

Earlier we argued that to understand better the effects of malnutrition on functioning, much needed to be investigated, especially about the effects of prenatal and early childhood malnutrition on performance during the school years. These results appeared to be important to people concerned with education and nutrition. If links could be shown between childhood nutrition and educational performance, not only would the efficiency of educational investments benefit from actions to remove nutritional impairment, but also integrated intervention policies aiming at increasing the child's opportunities for education would prove more efficient in terms of allocation of total resources. This was the starting place for the Berkeley Project on Education and Nutrition.

In Chapter 3 we present the results of a careful and complex analysis using data from the INCAP longitudinal study to find out how prenatal and early childhood nutrition—in combination with other socioenvironmental factors of the family and village—affect children's growth, health, verbal development, and school performance. These analytical models show that children's height was indeed affected by nutritional intake combined with the ability to use the nutrients, and that size of child could be used as a proxy measure of the whole history of the child's past nutrition and health. These are strong and significant results, which imply that improved nutritional status can affect children's future opportunities. It is also shown that taller children are more likely to be farther advanced in verbal development, and more likely to attend school at an earlier age.

These results are important for development planning, enabling planners to trace the effects of continuing food intake (in combination with environmental and family factors) to outcomes important for the children's lives. If such results could be combined with other important information about family economics, work, and perceptions of the economic utility of children (with resulting effects on the number of children in a family), it would be possible to understand more fully the range of opportunities for children in the rural village setting. It would then be possible to relate the effects of improved nutritional intake, health, and educational opportunity to the actual functioning of children in the villages.

Moreover, if the intergenerational effects of education could be measured in economic terms (by the impact of adult literacy on economic productivity), then school attainment could be related to economic productivity benefits. Development planners then could take into account benefits achieved by one sector on another— described by economists as "positive externalities." Better nutrition for children—leading to improved growth, stamina, verbal development, school attainment, work performance, and, ultimately, adult efficiency—combined with appropriate levels of land accessibility and school quality—would enhance lives beyond the gains expected by changes in nutrition alone.

We were encouraged, therefore, to discover that not only were data available to study the longitudinal effects of nutrition on growth, development, and school performance, but also that the great variety of data collected by INCAP and RAND permitted us to investigate relationships between children's school and work activities, parental economic productivity and literacy, and parental literacy and perceptions about desirable family size. In other words, the data let us look at the children's lives in the socioeconomic context of family and village and examine (1) how immediate needs for children's help affect a family's decisions about giving this up to meet the greater desirability of literacy; (2) the effects on adults' economic productivity of attained literacy; (3) the effect on the perceptions of economic utility of parent's literacy.

These three sets of important relationships are explored in Chapters 4, 5, and 6. Using cross-sectional data as well as the findings of Chapter 3, in Chapter 4 we examine variables that may explain parental decisions about sending children to school. Also Chapter 4 looks at the way nutritional status, parental literacy, family background, and economic conditions affect educational enrollment and achievement. Using Wilson's findings described in Chapter 3, attained height becomes the proxy measure for children's past nutritional and health status. Relationships between prior nutrition and health and school achievement are seen to vary by village and by type of economic activity of the family, indicating that while the opportunity for schooling may be available to all, those children who attend school will do so because parents can spare their work, or because parents value highly the benefits of schooling in the long term in relation to short-term costs. Within these constraints of the family as decision-makers, we then investigate whether attained height (a proxy for prior health and nutrition) does appear to affect the likelihood of school enrollment and achievement.

In Chapter 5 family agricultural production is related to land holdings, type of production, and farmer's literacy. Education is tested in how it affects the ability of farmers to choose the best combination of production factors, to introduce modern crops and chemical inputs, and to obtain, on the whole, higher levels of land and labor productivity. The estimation of a production function for different groups of farmers, according to their level of market integration, provided information about the influence of literacy and also about how an additional year of schooling affects the percentage increase of agricultural production. Derived values of marginal productivity of labor inputs indicate the magnitude of underemployment observed among farmers; this provides the basis for speculation about the influence of using children's work on the observed magnitude of underemployment among small farmers.

In Chapter 6 individual fertility behavior and desires are related to perceived economic need for children, family economic activity, and literacy of the heads of the household. These results allow us to see how increasing schooling and literacy, and altering other background factors of the female and male head of household, may affect attitudes toward family size and fertility and, ultimately, the future opportunity of each child in the rural setting.

References

ALEXANDER, LEIGH, and JOHN SIMMONS. *The Determinants of School Achievement in Developing Countries.* Washington, D.C.: World Bank Working Paper #201, 1975.

ANTONOV, A. N. "Children Born During the Siege of Leningrad in 1942." *Journal of Pediatrics* 30(1947):250–259.

BARNES, R. H., A. U. MOORE, I. M. REID, and W. G. POND. "Effect of Food Deprivation on Behavioral Patterns." In *Malnutrition, Learning, and Behavior,* edited by Nevin Scrimshaw and John Gordon. Cambridge, Mass.: MIT Press, 1968.

BIRCH, HERBERT. "Functional Effects of Fetal Malnutrition." In *Annual Progress in Child Psychiatry and Child Development,* edited by Stella Chess and Alexander Thomas, pp. 96–113. New York: Brunner/Mazel, 1972.

BIRCH, HERBERT, and JOAN DYE GUSSOW. *Disadvantaged Children: Health, Nutrition, and School Failure.* New York: Harcourt, Brace, and World, 1970.

BROZEK, JOSEF. *Behavioral Effects of Energy and Protein Deficits.* Washington, D.C.: U.S. Department of Health, Education and Welfare, NIH Publication #79-1906, 1979.

BUTZ, WILLIAM, and JEAN-PIERRE HABICHT. "The Effects of Nutrition and Health on Fertility: Hypotheses, Evidence, and Interventions." In *Population and Development: The Search for Selective Interventions,* edited by Ronald Ridker. Baltimore: The Johns Hopkins University Press, 1976.

CHAVEZ, ADOLFO, and CELIA MARTINEZ. "Behavioral Effects of Undernutrition and Food Supplementation." In *Behavioral Effects of Energy and Protein Deficits,* edited by Josef Brozek. Washington, D.C.: NIH Publication #79-1906, 1979.

CHAVEZ, ADOLFO, CELIA MARTINEZ, and TAMARA YASCHINE. "The Importance of Nutrition and Stimulation on Child Mental and Social Development." In *Early Malnutrition and Mental Development,* edited by Joaquin Cravioto, Leif Hambraeus, and Bo Vahlquist. Uppsala, Sweden: Almquist and Wiksell, 1974.

CHAVEZ, ADOLFO, CELIA MARTINEZ, and TAMARA YASCHINE. "Nutrition, Behavioral Development, and Mother Child Interaction in Young Rural Children." *Federation Proceedings* 34(1975):1574.

CHEN, LINCOLN, MYANOUR RAHMAN, and A. M. SARDER. "Epidemiology and Causes of Death among Children in a Rural Area of Bangladesh." *International Journal of Epidemiology* 9, 1 (1980).

CHEN, LINCOLN, EMDADUL HUQ, and SANDRA HUFFMAN. "A Prospective Study of the Risk of the Diarrheal Diseases according to Nutritional Status of Children." Unpublished paper. 1980.

CHEN, LINCOLN, ALAUDDIN CHOWDURY, and SANDRA HUFFMAN. "Anthropometric Assessment of Energy-Protein Malnutrition and Subsequent Risk of Mortality among Preschool Aged Children." *American Journal of Clinical Nutrition* 32, 8 (1980).

CHRISTIANSEN, N., L. VUORI, J. O. MORA, and M. WAGNER. "Social Environment as It Relates to Malnutrition and Mental Development." In *Early Malnutrition and Mental Development*, edited by Joaquin Cravioto, Leif Hambraeus, and Bo Vahlquist. Uppsala, Sweden: Almquist and Wiksell, 1974.

COATE, DOUGLAS, and DOV CHERNICKOVSKY. *An Economic Analysis of the Diet, Growth, and Health of Young Children in the United States*. Washington, D.C.: National Bureau of Economic Research, Working Paper #416, 1979.

COHN, ELCHANAN. *The Economics of Education*. Cambridge, Mass.: Ballinger, 1979.

COLDOUGH, CHRISTOPHER. *Primary Schooling and Economic Development: A Review of the Evidence*. Washington, D.C.: World Bank Staff Working Paper #399, 1980.

CRAVIOTO, J., and E. R. DELICARDIE. "The Effect of Malnutrition on the Individual." In *Nutrition, National Development, and Planning*, edited by Alan Berg, Nevin Scrimshaw and David Call. Cambridge, Mass.: MIT Press, 1973.

CRAVIOTO, J., and E. R. DELICARDIE. "Intersensory Development of School-Age Children." In *Malnutrition, Learning and Behavior*, edited by Nevin Scrimshaw and John Gordon. Cambridge, Mass.: MIT Press, 1968.

DOBBING, JOHN. "Nutrition and Brain Development." In *Present Knowledge in Nutrition*, 4th ed. New York: The Nutrition Foundation, 1976.

DOBBING, JOHN, and J. L. SMART. "Vulnerability of Developing Brain and Behaviour." *British Medical Bulletin* 30(1974):164-168.

DRILLIEN, C. M. "A Longitudinal Study of the Growth and Development of Prematurely and Maturely Born Children." *Archives of Diseases of Childhood* 36(1960):232-240.

EDWARDS, LINDA, and MICHAEL GROSSMAN. *Adolescent Health, Family Background and Preventive Medical Care*. Cambridge, Mass.: National Bureau of Economic Research Working Paper #398, 1979.

FRANKOVA, S. "Interaction Between Early Malnutrition and Stimulation in Animals." In *Early Malnutrition and Mental Development*, edited by Joaquin Cravioto, Leif Hambraeus, and Bo Vahlquist. Uppsala, Sweden: Almquist and Wiksell, 1974.

FRANKOVA, S. "Nutritional and Psychological Factors in the Development of Spontaneous Behavior in the Rat." In *Malnutrition, Learning, and Behavior*, edited by Nevin Scrimshaw and John Gordon. Cambridge, Mass.: MIT Press, 1968.

FRANKOVA, S., and R. H. BARNES. "Effect of Malnutrition in Early Life on Avoidance Conditioning and Behavior of Adult Rats." *Journal of Nutrition* 96(1968):485-493.

GRAVES, P. L. "Nutrition, Infant Behavior, and Maternal Characteristics: A Pilot Study in West Bengal, India." *The American Journal of Clinical Nutrition* 29(March 1976):305-319.

KLEIN, R. E., C. YARBROUGH, R. E. LASKY, and J. P. HABICHT. "Correlations of Mild to Moderate Protein-Calorie Malnutrition among Rural Guatemalan Infants and Preschool Children." In *Early Malnutrition and Mental Development*, edited by Joaquin Cravioto, Leif Hambraeus, and Bo Vahlquist. Uppsala, Sweden: Almquist and Wiksell, 1974.

KLEIN, R. E., M. IRWIN, P. E. ENGLE, and C. YARBROUGH. "Malnutrition and Mental Development in Rural Guatemala: An Applied Cross-Cultural Research Study." In *Advances in Cross-Cultural Psychology*, edited by N. Warren. New York: Academic Press, 1977.

KLEIN, R. E., M. IRWIN, J. TOWNSEND, et al. "The Effects of Food Supplementation on Cognitive Development and Behavior among Rural Guatemalan Children." In *Behavioral Effects of Energy and Protein Deficits*, edited by Josef Brozek. Washington, D.C.: NIH Publication #79-1906, 1979.

KNUDSEN, ODIN, and PASQUALE SCANDIZZO. *Nutrition and Food Needs in Developing Countries*. Washington, D.C.: World Bank Staff Working Paper #328, 1979.

LATHAM, MICHAEL. "Nutritional Problems in the Labor Force and Their Relation to Economic Development." In *Nutrition and Agricultural Development*, edited by Nevin Scrimshaw and Moíses Béhar. New York: Plenum Press, 1976.

LAVALLEE, M., P. DASEN, J. RETSCHITZKI, M. REINHARDT, and C. MEYLAN. "Subclinical Malnutrition and Sensorimotor Development in a Rural Area of the Ivory Coast." In *Behavioral Effects of Energy and Protein Deficits*, edited by Josef Brozek. Washington, D.C.: NIH Publication #79-1906, 1979.

LEVITSKY, D. A. "Malnutrition and Animal Models of Cognitive Development." In *Nutrition and Mental Function*, edited by George Serban. New York: Plenum Press, 1975.

LEWIS, OSCAR. *The Children of Sanchez*. New York: Random House, 1961.

MCFARLANE, HYLTON. "Nutrition and Immunity." In *Nutrition Reviews, Present Knowledge in Nutrition*. New York: Nutrition Foundation, 1976.

MCKAY, H., and L. SINISTERRA. "Intellectual Development of Malnourished Preschool Children in Programs of Stimulation and Nutritional Supplementation." In *Early Malnutrition and Mental Development*, edited by Joaquin Cravioto, Leif Hambraeus, and Bo Vahlquist. Uppsala, Sweden: Almquist and Wiksell, 1974.

MCKAY, HARRISON, LEONARDO SINISTERRA, ARLENE MCKAY, HERNANDO GOMEZ, and PASCUALA LLOREDA. "Improving Cognitive Ability in Chronically Deprived Children." *Science 200*: April 21, 1978.

MILNER, R. D. G. "Protein-Calorie Malnutrition." In *Present Knowledge in Nutrition*, edited by D. M. Hegsted. New York: The Nutrition Foundation, 1976.

MÖNCKEBERG, F. "Effect of Early Marasmic Malnutrition on Subsequent Physical and Psychological Development." In *Malnutrition, Learning and Behavior*, edited by Nevin Scrimshaw and John Gordon. Cambridge, Mass.: MIT Press, 1968.

MORA, C., M. WAGNER, L. DE NAVARRO, N. CHRISTIANSEN and M. G. HERRERA. "Nutritional Supplementation and the Outcome of Pregnancy." *American Journal of Clinical Nutrition 32*(February 1979):455–462.

MORA, J. O., A. AMEZQUITA, L. CASTRO, N. CHRISTIANSEN, J. CLEMENT-MURPHY, L. F. COBOS, H. D. CREMER, et al. "Nutrition, Health and Social Factors Related to Intellectual Performance." *World Review of Nutrition and Dietetics 10*(1974):205–236.

POLLITT, ERNESTO. *Poverty and Malnutrition in Latin America: Early Childhood Intervention Programs*. New York: Praeger Publishers, 1979.

POPKIN, BARRY, and MARISOL LIM-YBANEZ. "Nutrition and School Achievement." Forthcoming in *Social Science and Medicine*.

PRESCOTT, J. W., M. S. READ, AND D. B. COURSIN. *Brain Function and Malnutrition*. New York: John Wiley and Sons, 1975.

PSACHAROPOULOS, GEORGE. *Returns to Education: An International Comparison*. San Francisco: Jossey-Bass, Inc., 1973.

READ, MERRILL S. "Lessons from Latin American Studies of Malnutrition and Behavior." In *Behavioral Effects of Energy and Protein Deficits*, edited by Josef Brozek. Washington, D.C.: NIH Publication #79-1906, 1979.

REUTLINGER, SHLOMO. *The Prevalence of Calorie Deficit Diets in Developing Countries*. Washington, D.C.: World Bank Staff Working Paper #374, 1980.

RICCIUTI, HENRY. "Adverse Social and Biological Influences on Early Development." In *Ecological Factors in Human Development*, edited by Harry McGurk. New York: North-Holland, 1977.

RICHARDSON, STEPHEN. "Severity of Malnutrition in Infancy and Its Relation to Later Intelligence." *Behavioral Effects of Energy and Protein Deficits*. Washington, D.C.: National Institutes of Health, 1979.

ROSENBERG, IRWIN H., NOEL SOLOMON, and DOUGLAS LEVIN. "Interaction of Infection and Nutrition: Some Practical Concerns." *Ecology of Food and Nutrition* 4(1976):203–206.

ROSENZWEIG, MARK, and EDWARD BENNETT. "How Plastic is the Nervous System?" *The Comprehensive Handbook of Behavioral Medicine*. New York: SP Medical and Scientific Books, 1980.

ROSENZWEIG, MARK R. "Animal Models for Effects of Brain Lesions and for Rehabilitation." In *Recovery of Function: Theoretical Consideration for Brain Injury Rehabilitation*, edited by Paul Bach-y-Rita. Bern: Hans Huber, 1980.

SECKLER, DAVID. "Small But Healthy: A Crucial Hypothesis in the Theory, Measurement and Policy of Malnutrition." Unpublished paper. 1980.

SELOWSKY, MARCELO. *The Economic Dimensions of Malnutrition in Young Children*. Washington, D.C.: World Bank Staff Working Paper #294, 1978.

SELOWSKY, MARCELO. "Nutrition, Health, and Education: The Economic Significance of Complementarities at Early Ages." Unpublished paper. 1980.

SHARMA, R. C., and C. L. SAPRA. *Wastage and Stagnation in Primary and Middle Schools in India*. New Delhi: National Council of Educational Research and Training, 1969.

STEIN, Z., M. SUSSER, G. SAENGER, and F. MOROLLA. *Famine and Human Development: The Dutch Hunger Winter of 1944/45*. New York: Oxford University Press, 1975.

STEIN, Z., and M. SUSSER. "Prenatal Nutrition and Subsequent Development." In *The Epidemiology of Prematurity*, edited by Dwayne Reed and Fiona Stanley. Baltimore: Urban and Schwarzenberg, 1977.

SOURANDER, P., A. SIMI, and M. HALBIA. "Malnutrition and Morphological Development of the Nervous System." In *Early Malnutrition and Mental Development*, edited by Joaquin Cravioto, Leif Hambraeus, and Bo Vahlquist. Uppsala, Sweden: Almquist and Wiksell, 1974.

SRINVASAN, T. N. *Malnutrition: Some Measurement and Policy Issues*. Washington, D.C.: World Bank Staff Working Paper #373, 1980.

SUKHATME, P. V. "Economics of Nutrition." *Indian Journal of Agricultural Economics 32*, no. 3, 1977.

TANNER, J. M. "Population Differences in Body Size, Shape, and Growth Rate: A 1976 View." *Archives of Diseases of Childhood* 51(1976):1–2.

TANNER, J. M. *Fetus into Man*. Cambridge, Mass.: Harvard University Press, 1978.

WEINBERG, WARREN, SUSAN DIETZ, ELISABETH PENICK, and WILLIAM MCALISTER. "Intelligence, Reading Achievement, Physical Size, and Social Class." *Journal of Pediatrics* 85(1974), 4:482–489.

WINICK, MYRON. *Malnutrition and Brain Development*. New York: Oxford University Press, 1976.

WINIKOFF, BEVERLY, AND GEORGE BROWN. "Nutrition, Population, and Health: Theoretical and Practical Issues." *Social Science and Medicine 14C*(1980):171–176.

WORLD BANK. *World Bank Development Report*. New York: Oxford University Press, 1980.

WORLD FOOD AND NUTRITION STUDY. *The Potential Contribution of Research*. Washington, D.C.: National Academy of Sciences, 1977.

Chapter 2

THE GUATEMALAN EXPERIMENT—THE VILLAGES AND THE DATA*

by Members of the Berkeley Project on Education and Nutrition

Our analytical work was based on the study carried out in four rural communities in Eastern Guatemala by INCAP (1969–1978) and by RAND (1974–1975). Before we can discuss our own work, therefore, we must sketch the setting in Guatemala where the nutrition experiment took place, the experiment itself, and the data base assembled by the INCAP and RAND teams.

We begin by describing the villages, including some background on geography and demography; agricultural production; economic factors, including poverty; and education. Since the villages were chosen to be as similar as possible, we will point out not only apparent similarities but also characteristics for which important differences are observed. Next follows a description of the nutritional experiment (including treatment and control groups) and the manner in which it was carried out. Finally, we discuss the data collection upon which our analysis was based.

The Four Villages

Approximately one hundred villages were surveyed in the late 1960s; these four were chosen because of similarity in such impor-

---

* This chapter was drawn from material assembled by members of the Berkeley Project on Education and Nutrition. Further information on the villages appears in Chapters 3 to 6.

tant areas as economic factors, demographic composition, size, and ethnic makeup. Because, of course, it would be impossible to find four identical villages anywhere, in conducting analysis it is necessary to recognize and understand the differences in village characteristics—particularly so for a quasi-experimental* study in the natural setting such as is described here.

The nutritional-supplementation experiment and the related collection of data can be understood better when the reader has some background information about the four rural communities in Guatemala where the study took place. Here we shall give only a brief overview. Readers who seek more information will find a detailed and fascinating anthropological description in an article by Victor Mejía Pivaral (1972). Statistical treatment of data on the four villages is contained also in an unpublished report by Fraser and Sinay (1978). Table 2-1 gives a statistical picture of the villages.

Table 2-1   A Statistical Picture of the Four Villages[a]

	Village Number			
Measure	1	2	3	4
Population (approximate)	1200	1250	900	750
Elevation (in meters above sea level)	Approx. 800m	Approx. 800m	275m	Approx. 800m
Distance from Guatemala City	37km	58km	102km	56km
Distance from Highway	2km	4km	20km	9km
Average Family Income ($1 = 1 quetzal)	$531.4	$662.7	$489.2	$465.4
Average per Capita Income	$136.7	$167.5	$111.4	$ 88.7
Family Agricultural Income (includes both consumed and sold)	$170.9	$355.2	$263.8	$170.8
Family Nonagricultural Income	$360.5	$307.5	$225.4	$294.6

* A quasi-experiment is one in the natural setting where the experimenter cannot assign units to treatments at random. Here the villages (N = 4) were assigned at random, but individuals within villages were free to consume or not consume supplement.

Table 2-1 (continued)

Average Daily Wages	$.75	$.85	$.87	$.84
Father's Literacy	55%	49%	68%	44%
Mother's Literacy	51%	37%	35%	39%
Literacy of Males over 7 years	39%	30%	57%	32%
Literacy of Females over 7 years	36%	24%	29%	22%
School Participation, Boys 7–16	61%	35%	66%	52%
School Participation, Girls 7–16	55%	50%	55%	46%
Average Family Size	5.11	5.25	4.84	5.54
Completed Parity of Women 45–55	8.13	8.86	8.11	9.71
Child Mortality Rate: Children Died/Children Born	17%	23%	17%	20%
Housing: House Type (Scale 1, 2, 3, 4)	2.9	2.6	2.2	2.9
Water (public or private well)	100%	67.8%	64.2%	99.2%
Sanitation (some facilities)	14%	17%	23%	10%
Separate Kitchen	64%	61%	56%	77%
Male Heads of Family (N)	174	196	131	114
Principal Occupation of Male Heads: Agricultural Day Laborer	5%	7%	28%	3%
Farmer	80%	85%	57%	89%
Nonagricultural Day Laborer	4%	2%	1%	1%
Manufacturing	0%	0%	3%	0%
Merchant	1%	0%	2%	3%

Table 2-1 (continued)

Specialized Labor/Factory	5%	3%	4%	3%
Blue/White Collar Professional	5%	1%	2%	0%
No Occupation	0%	1%	1%	0%
Female Heads of Family (N)	179	153	133	109
Principal Occupation of Female Heads:				
Agricultural Day Laborer	0%	4%	2%	0%
Farmer	0%	5%	0%	1%
Domestic	4%	2%	2%	2%
Manufacturing	0%	0%	68%	0%
Merchant	6%	9%	4%	5%
Specialized Labor/Factory	2%	4%	2%	3%
No Occupation	86%	76%	20%	86%
Family Production Mode[b]				
Wage-Labor:				
(Percentage)	27%	20%	41%	18%
(Number)	55	44	70	22
Subsistence Farmer:				
(Percentage)	27%	19%	22%	39%
(Number)	55	43	38	47
Semi-Commercial Farmer:				
(Percentage)	27%	29%	12%	25%
(Number)	55	64	20	30
Commercial Farmer:				
(Percentage)	19%	32%	26%	19%
(Number)	39	71	44	23

[a] Several INCAP/RAND surveys were the sources of these measures. Since sample size varies according to timing and coverage, these measures may vary according to the questionnaire used.

[b] Wage-labor = no reported agricultural production; subsistence farmer = some agricultural production; semi-commercial farmer = agricultural production, some sold; commercial farmer = agricultural production, selling of production, and hiring wage-labor.

Geography/Demography

All the villages are located in the Department of El Progreso in the dry, mountainous area northeast of Guatemala City. Distances from the capital vary between 36 and 102 kilometers, but all suffer from the lack of direct public transportation from Guatemala City. Because roads are in relatively poor condition, traffic between the villages and outside communities is light. These villages, then, were seen as good choices for the longitudinal experiment, since patterns of life probably would remain more or less undisturbed.

The village center consists of the place where the small church and/or school are located. (The clinic and supplementation center built by INCAP also was located here.) There may be a small plaza, sometimes merely a widened place in the dirt road, with a simple store or flour mill located nearby. The main meeting place is the village well, where women and children congregate. Houses are located around this center on small roads and footpaths. Farm plots generally are located out of town, away from the communities.

Houses are built of local materials, usually with dirt floors and tile roofs (though now, since the earthquake in 1976, metal roofs often are found); walls are reed or adobe. Most of the houses are owned by the occupying family and consist of one or two rooms, generally following the Ladino custom of separating the kitchen from other rooms and sometimes locating it outdoors. Only Village 3 has electric power, but at the time of the survey fewer than half of its families had electricity at home. In two villages (1 and 4) water is piped to the communities, and there are public wells. In the others, a few households have their own wells, half use public wells, and another third must bring water from a nearby river. Sanitation (chiefly latrines) is almost nonexistent. More than half the families own radios and a few (10 percent) have sewing machines. House type (rated by materials used, and number of rooms) is a useful method of measuring wealth for Ladino families (Tumin, 1952). Since extended families often live in a combined household, it is not always possible to use house type as a measure of wealth, independent of the age of the family head.

The culture of all four villages is Ladino, indicating that the people speak Spanish and have adopted practices of the modern, rather than traditional, Indian culture. Most villagers are nominally Catholic, although an active Protestant group also exists in Village 1.

By the time she is 37, each mother has had, on the average, 5.7 children, and at the end of her childbearing years the average number is 8.6 children. Contraception is rarely used among the villagers, although a national radio campaign has created some awareness of its availability. Women have babies at close intervals and breast-feed them for long periods (see Chapter 6 for a fuller discussion of family-planning knowledge and practice).

The family living unit consists, on the average, of 5.2 persons with a child-mortality rate of 19 percent. Family diet is chiefly corn and beans; eggs, chicken, and pork from home-grown livestock; and occasionally fish, in one of the villages. Total energy intake in the home diet is limited. (This is an issue to be discussed in Chapter 3.)

Agricultural Production

The communities are primarily agricultural, with farming concentrated in five basic crops: corn and beans (food crops), tomatoes and chili (cash crops), and *maicillo* (animal feed). Other, less-important products include *ayoit* and yucca. The average farm plot is quite small (1.3 hectares) but families tend to have more than one plot. Total family landholdings average 2.8 hectares.

The rainy season comes between May and September. In April and May the soil is prepared; sowing takes place in late summer; and crops are harvested during the fall. During the busy seasons many family members join in farming activities. Climatic conditions are similar for the three villages which lie approximately 800 meters above sea level (Villages 1, 2, and 4); the fourth (Village 3), at 275 meters, gets less rain but has warmer temperatures. Also, the latter village differs from the others in being considerably farther from Guatemala City (104 km as against 36–58 km) but relatively close to a larger town in which some of the village children attend school.

Economic Factors and Poverty

Almost all (90 percent) male heads of families have agricultural occupations, including men who work as day laborers for other farmers. In the dry season some families leave the home villages to earn wages as harvesters. Most (80 percent) female heads of families do not work for money, except in one village where about three fourths of the women weave palm products; these are bought by merchants who sell them in Guatemala City.

Although the economy is chiefly agricultural, only a small proportion (17 percent) of families depend entirely on farming income.

Sales and salaried work yield a substantial amount of cash income; sales, wages, and income from such activities as small trade and arts and crafts add up to 60 percent of total income, on the average. (In most of the villages hiring labor seems to be a common practice.) Wage income alone accounts for about 40 percent of total income.

Average family income is about $550 per year; average annual income per capita (where data were available) is approximately $130. This is very low, even when compared to the Guatemalan per capita average of $910 (World Bank, 1980)—in itself relatively low compared to the averages of other Latin American countries.

Even among these four predominantly poor villages, substantial inequalities exist within each. In terms of land distribution, the upper quintile of farmers controls more than 40 percent of the land. As for total income, wages and other income sources compensated for a small part of the skewed distribution in land; but, even so, 5 percent of the wealthiest families received 25 percent of the income. The direct consequence of such unequal distribution of means of production and inequality in income is that a considerable number of families lie below the absolute poverty level, even when poverty is defined by local standards—about 35 percent of families in the study villages fall into this category.

Education

Literacy levels are low; less than half the villagers over age seven are literate, men more likely to be so than women. Those employed in nonagricultural activities are more likely to be literate than are agricultural workers. The ability to read and write is most important in getting work outside the villages; for example, young women who want to work in Guatemala City as domestics have a better chance at jobs if they can read, as do men who seek work in the modern sector outside the villages. More than half the villagers over age seven have finished no grades in school. Differences between males and females in numbers of grades passed is small, except in one community (Village 3) in which many more men than women have gone to school.

Each village has a primary school, consisting of three or four rooms, with desks, chairs, and blackboards as the sparse and only equipment. Children must provide their own books and supplies— and some cannot. First and second grades are in separate classrooms but there is doubling up for other grades. First grade usually has the largest enrollment; the combined fourth, fifth, and sixth have few children in attendance. Boys' involvement in school generally is higher than girls'.

Rural teachers are trained in rural pedagogical institutions, receiving poorer preparation than those destined to work in urban schools. Teachers in our four villages apparently vary in interest and commitment to their work, and some are frequently absent; some teachers commute daily to the villages from Guatemala City where they live. Communication between parents and teachers appears to depend on how involved the teachers themselves are in community life.

The school year runs from January through October, thereby competing with the demands of planting and harvest seasons; between March and June classes are held from 8 to 12 A.M. and from July to October from 8 to 12 and 2 to 4 P.M. Although children may start school at age seven, many do not begin until eight, nine, or even ten. It is common to repeat grades; of those children aged ten, about 70 percent still are in school but may not have advanced past first or second grade.

Although the Guatemalan national plan for education states that all children must attend school, in fact it is not compulsory in these rural communities where the family economy may depend on children's work. When still very young, children begin to help—girls preparing food, caring for younger siblings, and carrying water; boys helping the fathers work family farm plots. Children are almost completely in the care of mothers until school age, at which time fathers begin to make decisions about children's (especially boys') activities. In Chapter 4 we shall describe more fully what children do, including paid work. Such activities differ by village and play an important role in determining whether or not a child will attend school.

Description of the INCAP Experiment

In order to understand the purpose of the quasi-experiment carried out by INCAP in Guatemala and to recognize what, in retrospect, may have been certain design flaws, it is necessary to realize that this work was based on assumptions about malnutrition current during the 1960s.

During the 1950s and 1960s, protein-energy malnutrition was believed to be a serious problem, particularly in developing countries. Little was published, however, about the long-range effects of PEM (protein-energy malnutrition) because the literature dealt almost exclusively with the severest cases, in which most of the children affected were hospitalized and many of them died. Obviously, this group represents only a small percentage of the estimated half to two thirds of the children in the developing world alleged to be suffering chronic, mild-to-moderate PEM. Furthermore, because at that time it was believed that PEM came primarily from dietary protein deficiency, new high-protein foods were developed also, and ways were sought to distribute these to pregnant women and infants, who are the most vulnerable members of that population.

The design of the Guatemalan study was predicated on this assumption—that protein was indeed the limiting factor. However, by the 1970s, some scholars began to realize that PEM (except in certain isolated areas, for example, of Africa, where the diet consisted mainly of tuberous materials) was not due to primary protein deficiency but rather to low caloric intake. This makes the body use protein stores for energy rather than for building tissues. In other words, if total calories were adequate, then the available protein would suffice.

In order to determine the effect of chronic, mild-to-moderate PEM on mental development (specifically, cognitive performance during the preschool years), groups of Guatemalan children and pregnant women were given a high-protein supplement. A control group was to be given no supplementation. Study children were followed during the preschool years, and measured frequently in order to determine what effects the environment and the supplement might have on a host of outcome variables. Investigators hoped to learn whether mild-to-moderate protein-energy malnutrition resulted in impaired cognitive performance during preschool years. INCAP further hoped to follow these individuals through school years, adolescence, and adulthood to see whether the effects, if any, were permanent.

The investigation was three years in preparation, during which time investigators identified two paris of matched villages and carried out extensive anthropological and ethnographic surveys. The study itself began early in 1969, and data collection continued for eight years, until March 1977.

The population in each of one pair of villages was about 850 residents, in the other pair, approximately 500. Based on the assumption that protein was the operant deficiency, one village in each pair received nutritional intervention consisting of a high-protein substance called Atole; the other village was controlled. In order to help minimize the effect of intervention per se, control villages were provided with a nonprotein, low-caloric drink, Fresco. All villages received free preventive and curative outpatient medical services for the duration of the study.

Data were collected on growth, morbidity, home diet, family socioeconomic status, and measures of mental development. As we said earlier, the villages were chosen because they were similar in a number of characteristics though, of course, not identical.

In January 1969 supplementation centers opened in all four villages and data collection started. In Villages 2 and 4 the supplement was Atole, which contained 11.5 grams of high-quality protein and 163 kcal energy per 180 ml, 28 percent of which was derived from protein. The other two villages (1, 3) were provided with a low-energy beverage called Fresco, which contained no protein and only about one third (approximately 59 kcal/180 ml) of the energy concentration in Atole. In October 1971 vitamins, minerals, and fluoride were added to both supplements in order to guard against the possibility that average home diets of the study families might have been deficient in these elements. This obviously complicated the analysis because the amount of vitamins and minerals varied depending on both the home diet and the amount of supplements ingested.

Distribution of the supplement took place every day for two hours in the morning and two hours in the afternoon. Attendance at the centers was voluntary, and the supplement was available ad libitum to all members of the family. Since both supplements were liquid, it was possible to measure accurately the amount taken. Atole and Fresco intakes by pregnant mothers and children under age seven were measured daily and recorded to the nearest centiliter. Table 2-2 provides some information about the amount of supplement consumed.

When the project began in January 1969, the sample included all children under seven years and all pregnant and lactating women. The village census was updated quarterly, and a child who reached age seven was dropped from the sample. Newborn and immigrating children under age seven were added. The last children included, born by February 1973, brought the total sample to 1400. Only children born after January 1969 were included in the Berkeley analysis.

Table 2-2 Yearly Average of Supplement Consumed in Cl/Week by Year of Child's Life

	1	2	3	4	5	6	7
Fresco	5.925	24.552	58.426	95.639	134.609	154.742	188.408
	(9.412)	(29.257)	(59.299)	(82.085)	(94.212)	(102.880)	(102.718)
Atole	45.475	83.939	105.839	110.261	105.440	107.271	114.188
	(54.770)	(78.174)	(93.361)	(101.816)	(98.569)	(109.979)	(113.773)

Note: First number is mean, and standard deviations are shown in parentheses.

Consumption of supplement is measured in centiliters:

1 cl = 10 ml = 1/18 cup
1 cl of Atole = 9.05 calories (kcal) and .638 grams of protein
1 cl of Fresco = 3.27 calories and 0 grams of protein
1 cup of Atole = 163 calories
1 cup of Fresco = 59 calories

The INCAP Data Base for the Berkeley Study

Study Variables

1. *Amount of food consumed.* Supplementation was measurable with great accuracy and reliability, and home dietary surveys also were made in order to estimate total food intake (home diet plus supplement). In field investigations such as this, there is always a question as to whether supplement actually is supplementary or is merely a replacement. Therefore, for these data to be meaningful, they must be (a) analyzed in terms of total food consumed, and (b) an estimate should be made of the potential error of home dietary measurements. In this instance, 24-hour recall data were collected at three-month intervals. Mothers were questioned about the previous day's intake, and interviewers recorded information on dietary patterns for pregnant and lactating women, as well as for all children between 15 and 84 months of age. At INCAP headquarters in Guatemala City specific nutrient intake was computed from the food composition tables prepared for Latin America and summarized in terms of calories, total protein, animal protein, calcium, iron, vitamin A, vitamin C, niacin, riboflavin, and thiamine.

2. *Anthropometry.* Using standard anthropometric techniques, the children were examined at birth; at 15 days; and every three months thereafter up to 24 months; then every six months between 30 and 48 months; and yearly up to 84 months. Data were collected on nine variables. These included: supine length, total body weight, medial calf circumference, condylar breadth of femur, triceps, subscapular and medial calf skinfolds. In addition, dental-eruption data were collected, and radiographs were made of the left hand and wrist of study children at the beginning, and at times when the children were otherwise examined.

3. *Biomedical data.* Biomedical data collected during the study consisted of medical-care records; clinic information on attendance; and symptomatology, pregnancy, delivery, and perinatal information. For a subsample of the study population, delivery information included: Apgar Score, examination of the infant, determination of mother's milk production, gestational age of the child, and urinary urea/creatinine ratio-determinations in lactating mothers and in children.

4. *Morbidity surveys.* Morbidity data collection began in 1970 on children seven years old or less, and in pregnant and lactating

mothers. The morbidity survey was made by retrospective home interviews of mothers every two weeks. These interviews were summarized monthly for each subject.

5. *Social and economic indicators.* A limited amount of data on a number of family and economic social indicators were collected also, including qualitative ratings of the family house, parents' clothing, and mother's report of interaction with preschool children. These data were gathered in 1968, 1972, 1973, and 1974. In addition, a vast amount of socioeconomic, family, educational, and agricultural-production data were collected in 1974 in a more detailed study by RAND.

6. *Mental development.* A wide variety of assessment techniques was used to measure mental development, many of which were developed specifically for this study. Such measurements obviously varied with the age of the child at the time of testing.

a. *Infant assessment.* A composite infant scale was developed from four, widely used, standard psychomotor infant tests: the Bailey Scale of Psychomotor Development, the Cattell Infant Scale, the Merrill-Palmer Scale, and the Gesell Scale. In 1972 two other infant assessments were added. One of these was the Brazelton Neonatal Scale; the second, the Infant Cognitive Battery, was introduced to assess mental changes during the last half of the first year of life.

b. *Preschool assessment.* Within two weeks of their third, fourth, fifth, sixth, and seventh birthdays, children in the longitudinal study received the INCAP Pre-School Battery, composed of twenty-one tests. Twelve of the tests (developed in 1967 and 1968) assessed a variety of cognitive processes; and the remaining nine (developed between 1970 and 1971) examined other areas of presumed theoretical importance. Also included were recognized I.Q. tests such as the Stanford-Binet.

The RAND Data Base

In 1974 the RAND Corporation carried out an extensive study using questionnaires. This study included a determination of agricultural wealth and production, an opinion survey of the parents, and a questionnaire concerning the activities of children. These questionnaires—designed to answer questions not included in the main nutritional hypothesis—served as a rich resource for us to use in analyzing the data.

The following list includes all surveys collected by RAND in 1974 and 1975.

R03:   Retrospective Life History of Women (fertility history). Administered to all women between ages 15–49 ever united in a marriage-type union or ever a mother. Dates: September–December 1974 and March–July 1975.

R05:   Home Stimulation. Administered to all pregnant women or women with children under seven years old in the rural communities and under three years old in the semi-urban communities. Dates: October–August 1975.

R06:   Modernism. Administered to same sample as R05 above. Dates: October–August 1975.

R07:   Mother's Vocabulary. Administered to same sample as R05 above. Dates: October–August 1975.

R08:   Schooling Survey. Administered to same sample as R05 above. Dates: October–August 1975.

R09:   Time-Use of Women and Children. Administered to same sample as R05 above. Dates: Round 1—December 1975, Round 2—March 1975, Round 3—July 1975, Round 4—November 1975.

R10:   Income and Wealth in 1974. Administered to all heads of households in the rural areas and to heads of households with R05–R09, all farmers, and one quarter of the rest for the semi-urban sample. Dates: January–August 1975.

R10B: Community Price Survey. Administered to three key people in each community. Dates: September 1975.

R11:   Attitudes and Expectations of Women. Administered to same sample as R03 above for rural sample and one half of the R05–R09 sample plus one quarter of the wives of the male respondents to R10 questionnaire in the semi-urban areas. Dates: November 1975–March 1976.

R12:   Attitudes and Expectations of Men.
Administered to one half of the husbands of the R03 respondents, to one half of the single men in the R10 sample for the rural areas, and to one third of the husbands of the respondents to the R11 Questionnaire.
Dates: December 1975–May 1976.

R13:   Retrospective Life History of Men.
Administered to same sample as R12 above.
Dates: December 1975–May 1976.

R14:   Income and Wealth in 1975.
Administered to one quarter of the heads of households in each community.
Dates: December 1975–May 1976.

425:    Household Census.
Administered to all residents of each community.
Dates: January–February 1975.

For full information about these surveys see Corona (1978). We shall refer to information that we used from the RAND surveys by name and number in the chapters that follow.

References

ADAMS, RICHARD N. *Cultural Surveys of Panama–Nicaragua–Guatemala–El Salvador–Honduras*. Scientific Publication No. 33. Washington, D.C.: Pan American Sanitary Bureau, 1951.

ADAMS, RICHARD N. *Crucifixion by Power: Essays on Guatemalan National Social Structure*. Austin: University of Texas Press, 1970.

CORONA, HENRY L. *Codebook and User's Manual: INCAP-RAND Guatemala Survey*. Santa Monica: RAND Corporation, 1978.

FRASER, JANE, and ELIANA SINAY. Appendix to the Final Report of the Berkeley Project on Education and Nutrition, School of Education, University of California, 1978. Unpublished.

PIVARAL, VICTOR MEJÍA. "Caracteristicas Economicas y Socio-Culturales de Cuatro Aldeas Ladinas de Guatemala." *Guatemala Indigena VII*, 3, 1972.

TUMIN, MELVIN. *Caste in a Peasant Society*. Princeton, N.J.: Princeton University Press, 1952.

WORLD BANK. *World Development Report 1980*. Washington, D.C.: Oxford University Press, 1980.

Chapter 3

LONGITUDINAL ANALYSIS OF DIET, PHYSICAL GROWTH, VERBAL DEVELOPMENT, AND SCHOOL PERFORMANCE

by Alan B. Wilson

In this chapter we seek to estimate some of the complex inter-relationships among economic and cultural characteristics of families, components of children's diet, incidence of morbidity, physical growth, and cognitive development. An enormous litera-ture bearing on these relationships has accumulated. Jelliffe (1975), for example, compiled a bibliography of more than 3,000 titles of studies relating PCM (protein calorie malnutrition) to deficits in growth and functioning. Some of these, along with more recent studies, are mentioned in Chapter 1. Despite this wealth of material many of the linkages remain uncertain.

While there is consistent evidence that chronic protein-calorie malnutrition (PCM) leads to stunting—indeed stature often is taken as an index of nutritional status—the levels of protein in the diet that will facilitate growth are controversial. The protein in the home diet of the INCAP study children in Guatemala (about 11 percent usable protein) is considerably higher than both the requirements and safe levels prescribed by the World Health Organization (WHO) (1973) for children of the same age and weight. This has led interpreters of the INCAP data to construe the effects of the protein-rich supple-ment, Atole, to be an increment to energy consumption, thus spar-ing dietary protein for growth (cf. Klein, 1977; Engle *et al.*, 1979; Cronbach, 1980, pp. 230–231). Recently Chernichovsky and Coate

(1979)—analyzing the HANES survey of nutrition of children in the United States (among whom both calorie and protein intakes are, on the average, considerably above prescribed standards for children of their age and weight)—found substantial effects of variations in dietary protein upon growth in height and head circumference. This led them to query: "Could American mothers, who provide very high protein diets for their children in households at all levels of socioeconomic status, know more about what constitutes an adequate diet for their children than the experts do?"

Because consumption of Atole supplements in the INCAP study leads to considerable variation in dietary protein between children, we have a unique opportunity to examine the separate effects upon growth of variations in protein and calories.

Despite a burgeoning literature, and such widely accepted social policies as school lunch programs—which attest to or assume a causal relationship between undernutrition, early mental development, and school performance—the evidence is not unambiguous. Children with severe early undernutrition leading to clinical marasmus show subsequent, impaired mental functioning. Even moderate chronic PCM, resulting in stunting, is associated with lower scores on mental tests (Klein *et al.*, 1972). Yet whether this relationship is directly causal or is a consequence of the web of disadvantaging factors associated with PCM—the ecology of poverty—is open to question (Thompson and Pollitt, 1977; Ricciuti, 1977). Analyses that have been especially sensitive to the confounding effects of the environment of poverty, however, continue to find a substantial relationship between nutrition and mental development (Chavez, Martinez, and Yaschine, 1974; Christiansen, Vuori, Mora, and Wagner, 1974; Cravioto and DeLicardie, 1972; Richardson, 1976).

The effects of current diet upon school performance are even less well documented. Several studies find, though a few fail to do so, that even in relatively well nourished populations in the United States, temporary hunger—as opposed to malnutrition—may adversely affect attention, interest, and learning (Read, 1973, 1975; Pollitt, Gersovitz, and Garguilo, 1978). This fits with Latham and Cobos's (1971) suggestion that low energy leading to inactivity has short-term effects upon learning which can be cumulative, regardless of long-term nutritional status.

The longitudinal data from the INCAP study enable us to look at the effects of variations in recent diet upon school performance (as judged by teachers), while holding constant prior cumulative nutri-

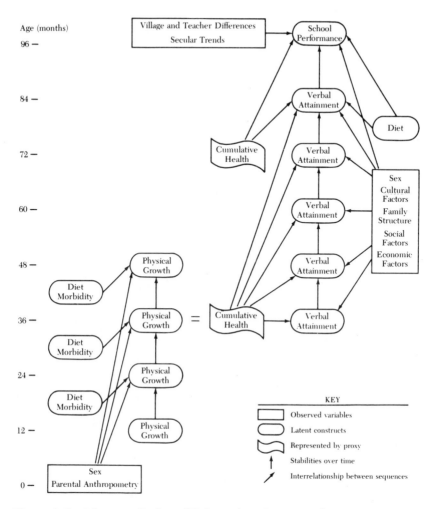

Figure 3-1 Schematic Outline of Relationships Investigated.

tional status, verbal attainment, and many background characteristics.

The sequence of topics which we shall address is sketched diagramatically in Figure 3-1. First we will describe the diets of children in the study villages to see how diets may differ between treatment groups. We will be particularly interested in whether provision of Atole by the INCAP field team acted to replace home diet or served as a genuine supplement.

Then we turn to the relationship between variations in diet, incidence of morbidity, and growth in weight and height among boys and girls during their second, third, and fourth years of life.

Finally, we will examine how early nutritional status affects cognitive development from age three through the first year of schooling at about age eight. Of particular interest here is the question as to whether current diet has any effect upon school performance among children with similar prior nutritional status and verbal development.

The analyses in this chapter are based on data from 824 children born between January 1969 (when INCAP started collecting data in the four study villages) and March 1972, and who had lived in one of the villages at any time during their first six years. This sample includes children who immigrated into the villages during the study period, or who left the village, or who died during their first six years. As in all field surveys, some data are missing for most variables. The largest source of such missing data appears for measurements after age five. The later cohorts of children (those born in 1972) did not attain age five until 1977 when data collection in the field had been discontinued.

From a close screening of censuses conducted periodically by INCAP, and once by RAND, we determined at what ages each of the 824 children lived in the villages; presumably these children would be available for data collection. Information on a few variables—age, sex, supplementation—was complete; at the other extreme, measurements of fathers' anthropometry were available for only about half of the cases. Coverage for most variables, however, ranged from 75–90 percent. The first half of this analysis—dealing with diet and growth during the first four years—is based on that subset of 512 children born in one of the villages who continued to live there at least until age three, which excluded most transients.

Diet and Physical Growth

Children's Home Diets and Supplements

Mothers in the Atole villages manifestly perceived the supplement to be good food, which it was; in Fresco villages supplement was (accurately) perceived as refreshment, but not as valuable food. By age three months infants in the Atole villages were consuming, on the average, over 50 kcal of energy from supplement; in the Fresco villages children at that age consume less than 3 kcal per day on the average. By age 18 months supplements comprised over 16 percent of the total diet of children in the Atole villages, as contrasted with

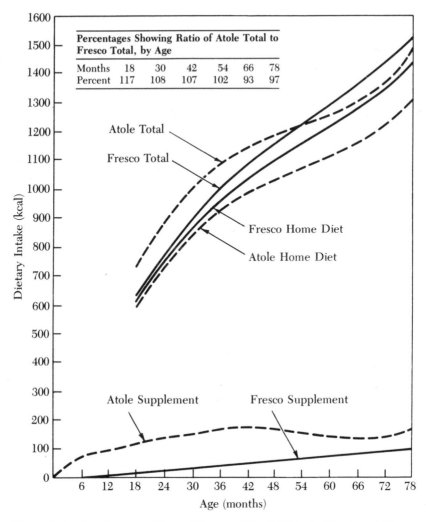

Percentages Showing Ratio of Atole Total to Fresco Total, by Age					
Months 18	30	42	54	66	78
Percent 117	108	107	102	93	97

Atole Total

Fresco Total

Fresco Home Diet

Atole Home Diet

Atole Supplement   Fresco Supplement

Figure 3-2 Supplements, Home Diets, and Total Diets by Treatment Group and Age: 0 to 84 Months.

but 2 percent of the diet of children in the Fresco villages. Average daily consumption in kcal units of supplement, home diet, and of the resultant total diets of children in the two groups of villages is shown graphically in Figure 3-2.*

---

* This and subsequent graphs of weight and height by age are smoothed by fitting a logarithmic term and polynomials of up to the sixth degree. Each curve for the longitudinal sample closely fits the raw data as indicated by values of R^2 greater than 0.999. The curve fitting was undertaken mainly to help interpolate between discrete ages when measurements were taken, and to allow for some sampling variability that resulted from missing data.

While children in the Atole villages, from shortly after birth through the first four years, consume substantially more supplement than those in the Fresco villages, home diets, on the average, are smaller at all ages for Atole-supplemented children. The availability of supplement, in addition to increasing total dietary intake, appears to replace a portion of home diet. We cannot measure directly how much these particular children would have eaten at home in the absence of intervention, but several bits of evidence do suggest that, prior to the intervention, the nutritional status of the population in the Atole villages was at least as good as that in the Fresco villages. First, there was no significant difference between the heights of parents in the Atole and Fresco villages, though both fathers and mothers in the Atole villages had significantly larger head circumferences. Second, records of the home diets of mothers during the third trimester of pregnancy during the project period show a steady decline of home diets in the Atole villages. There, mothers of children born in 1969 through 1971 were eating more at home than were pregnant mothers in the Fresco villages; toward the end of the project period, mothers in Atole villages were eating less at home than their counterparts in Fresco villages. Third, in a base-line study (conducted in 1968) of children's anthropometry in the study villages, very few significant differences showed up between children in the villages that would subsequently be offered Atole and those to be assigned Fresco. But then, too, differences in head circumferences systematically favored children in the Atole villages. (Selected data from this base-line study describing weights and heights of the cross-sectional sample in 1968 are displayed for comparative purposes in Figures 3-4 through 3-7.)

A significant part of the home diet of children during their first two years of life is omitted from our tally: the food derived from nursing. On the average, mothers continued to lactate for 18 months in these villages. In this regard, also, the villages differ. During the study period 61 percent of the mothers are still nursing babies at age 18 months in the Fresco villages; in the Atole villages only 43 percent of the mothers continue to lactate.

The introduction of this "free good," the Atole supplement, seems to have had three gross effects on children's diets in these villages: replacing a portion of home diet, causing mothers to wean children earlier, and enhancing children's total energy consumption.

Measurement of Home Diets.   As indicated in Chapter 2, data on children's home diets were elicited (at periodic intervals, beginning at age 15 months) by asking mothers to recall their children's consumption on the previous day. This sequence of observations has been averaged to generate six annual estimates of daily home diets at ages 18, 30, 42, 54, 66, and 78 months. For example, the diet reported at 18 months is average with the reports for 15 and 21 months. Thus three measures were used to generate each point estimate. Although the use of three reports should somewhat improve the reliability of measurement, the potential sources of error are substantial. Aside from the fallibility of parental recall, and inevitable errors of transcription and translation from tables of food values, these three reports are used to represent average (mid-point) consumption for 365 days. Given real variability in day-to-day consumption, the sampling error is potentially the largest component of error variance. The contrasts between mean diets of the children in Atole and Fresco villages, however, remain consistent from year to year and, because based on fairly large samples, are highly significant statistically.

Treatment Effects on Protein Consumption. We have seen that total energy intake during the first four years is somewhat larger in Atole than in Fresco villages (about 15 percent larger at age 18 months). This is due to the greater consumption of supplement in the Atole villages. Even this difference at 18 months may be exaggerated because of earlier weaning of children in the Atole villages. Because of the very high protein content of Atole, the contrast between groups in consumption of protein is much more pronounced. This contrast is displayed in Figure 3-3.

The protein value of the home diets of children in the four villages is similar—about 11 percent. Recall, however, that the Atole supplement contains 27 percent usable protein, while Fresco has none. As a result of consuming Atole, the total diet of children in the Atole villages at 18 months has 45 percent more protein than does that of their compeers in the Fresco villages.

At 18 months in the Fresco villages children weighing an average of 8.37 kg, consuming 16.25 gr of protein per day, are half again over WHO recommended levels; in the Atole villages at 8.87 kg, and consuming 23.75 gr of protein per day, children are over double the WHO recommended levels.

The largest effect of the nutritional invervention upon children's diets in these villages has been to increase the amount and proportion of protein in the diet in the Atole villages; the enhancement of total energy intake is more modest.

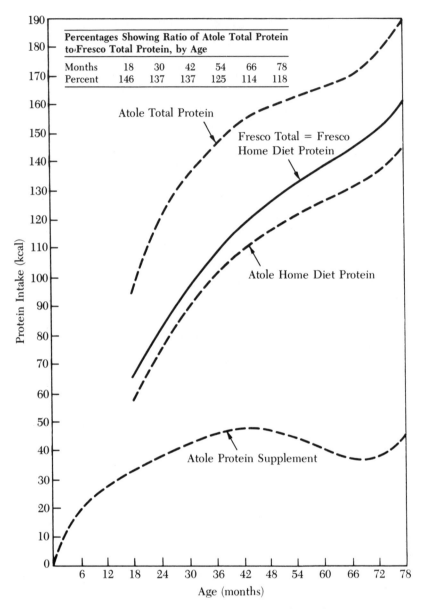

Percentages Showing Ratio of Atole Total Protein to Fresco Total Protein, by Age						
Months	18	30	42	54	66	78
Percent	146	137	137	125	114	118

Figure 3-3 Dietary Protein by Treatment Group and Age from Home Diets, Supplements, and Total.

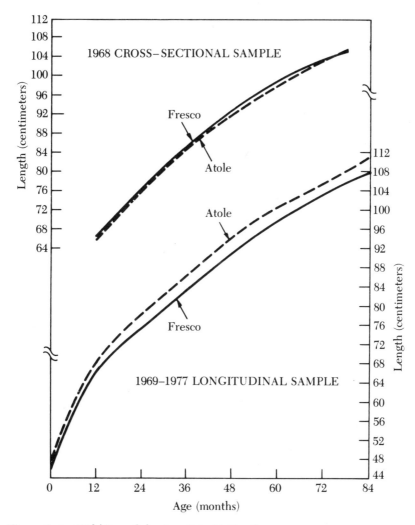

Figure 3-4 Girls' Length by Age: 0 to 84 Months.

Patterns of Physical Growth by Sex and Treatment

Average growth curves for the same 512 children whose diets have just been discussed are presented in the lower portions of Figures 3-4 through 3-7. The upper part of each figure contains growth curves of samples of children measured in 1968 in the study villages. The curves for the longitudinal sample, based on the same children at different ages (though only the earlier cohorts are represented by measurements after 54 months), closely fit the observed means. The

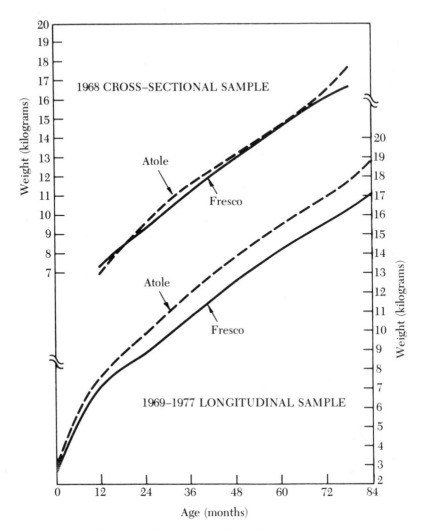

Figure 3-5 Girls' Weight by Age: 0 to 84 Months.

cross-sectional curves, on the other hand, being based on samples of children who were of different ages at the same time, are fitted through data points that are more widely scattered. (The fitted curves, containing high-order polynomials, also are more irregular.)

In the lower portions of each figure the advantage of children enjoying the Atole supplement is clear and consistent. In the 1968 cross-sectional base-line survey shown in the upper portions, the estimated growth curves, though irregular, are close together and do not show a systematic advantage for one village group over the

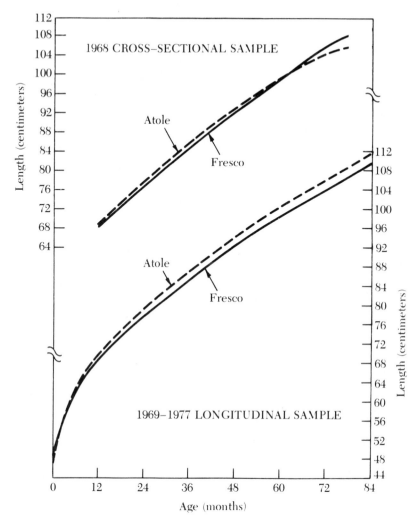

Figure 3-6 Boys' Length by Age: 0 to 84 Months.

other. The most apparent difference in these base-line data is that boys in Atole villages seem slightly heavier than boys in Fresco villages. This once again is congruent with our prior observation that the home diets of children in Atole villages were at least as ample as those in Fresco villages before the intervention, and that the Atole supplement in part replaced home diet.

In Figure 3-8 we have superimposed the weight curves for girls (from Figure 3-5) onto a chart of U.S. percentile norms (USNCHS, 1976). This detail points up the striking deceleration of growth

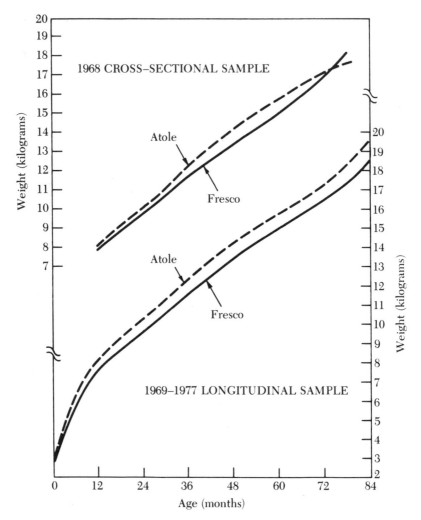

Figure 3-7 Boys' Weight by Age: 0 to 84 Months.

between the third and ninth month of life—more rapid and severe in Fresco than in Atole villages. While both groups fall below the fifth U.S. percentile norm by the age of 12 months, girls in Atole villages show a degree of recovery during their first year, by age three recovering to almost the tenth percentile. Girls in Fresco villages stay well below the fifth percentile and remain parallel to it thereafter.

The striking differences in patterns of growth between the treatment villages, compared with the small and inconsistent differences before the intervention, fit the interpretation that, despite some

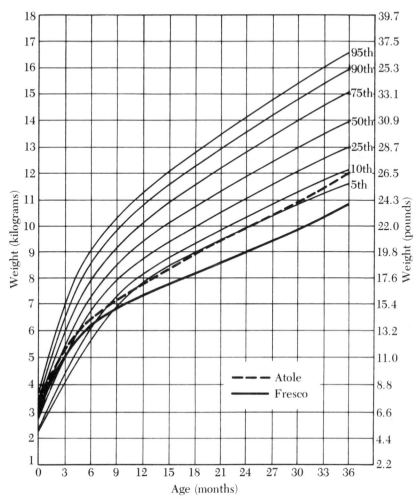

Figure 3-8 Girls' Weight by Age and Treatment Compared to U.S. Percentile Norms: 0 to 36 Months.

replacement of home diet, the availability of Atole did promote growth in both weight and height.*

But this gross effect does not clearly indicate whether the increment in total energy consumption in the Atole villages is sufficient to release enough already available protein to permit the observed growth, or whether growth results from the increased proportion of

---

* Analyzing the data as a randomized experiment—with villages nested in treatments, having only four cases (village means)—one finds significant treatment effects at each age level for both weight and height.

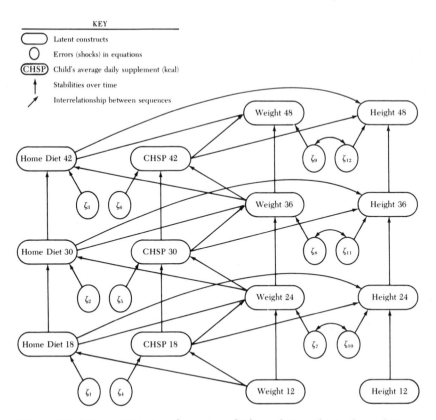

Figure 3-9 Home Diet, Supplement, and Physical Growth: Outline of Structural Relations among Endogenous Variables.

protein in the diets of these undernourished children. By prevailing standards the limiting factor in the children's home diets is an overall shortage of calories. Indeed, the actual quantity of protein in the home diets of children in the Fresco villages through their sixth year substantially exceeds what are considered safe levels for children of average size in the United States.

Home Diet, Supplements, and Physical Growth

If it were true that the total caloric value in Atole leads to extra growth among these children who, for the most part, already receive more than enough protein, one would anticipate that variations in growth among children would be similarly affected by variations in home diet and in supplementation.

Structural Model.   To estimate these effects we have developed a longitudinal model specifying hypothesized relations among four developmental sequences: home diet and supplementation at 18, 30, and 42 months; weight and height at 12, 24, 36, and 48 months; and 21 other exogenous variables. Figure 3-9 shows the main structural relations among the endogenous variables—the diet and growth sequences. Vertical arrows represent the "stabilities" in each sequence; for example, those who are taller at age 24 months can be expected to be taller at 36 months. The transverse arrows represent interrelationships between sequences. We allow for the likelihood that prior weight may influence the usual amount of food consumed. In turn, our hypothesis holds that both home diet and supplementation affect increases in weight and stature at the next time period.

A full glossary of acronyms used to represent names of variables can be found at the end of this chapter. In Figure 3-9 HT stands for height—actually supine length—in centimeters; CHSP represents a child's average daily supplement in kcal units. The numeric suffixes to these acronyms indicate the child's age in months.

The 21 additional exogenous variables are not shown in the path diagram. To include them graphically would yield a dense maze of crisscrossing arrows. These variables are indicated, however, by their acronyms in the structural equation—which corresponds to the path diagram, in Figure 3-10—and in the following tables which present the estimated coefficients. A mother's attendance at the supplementation center (MAATT) during the year, for example, may affect the average daily consumption of supplement by the child during the same year; mother's attendance at the center, per se, will not directly affect growth or home diet. If the mother is still lactating when the child is 18 months old (LACT18), this will affect the amount of other food the child usually eats, and may directly affect the child's growth during the second year of life. Diarrhea (CHD-IAR) and other morbidity (MORBOTH) may affect both diet and growth during each period. Other exogenous variables will be discussed substantively, in connection with numeric estimates of their effects.

Error Terms. The full model also specifies several sources of potential error. Each of the 12 simultaneous equations allows for unexplained variance in the dependent variable, represented by the zetas in Figures 3-9 and 3-10. This, of course, is standard in regression and structural equation models. In addition, however (as shown in the path diagram), because of the possibility that unmeasured factors might simultaneously affect growth in weight and height, errors in the equations may be correlated. This departs from the usual assumption of uncorrelated errors in equations.

	CHHD18	CHHD30	CHHD42	CHSP18	CHSP30	CHSP42	WT24	WT36	WT48	HT24	HT36	HT48		
CHHD18	1	0	0	0	0	0	0	0	0	0	0	0		η_1
CHHD30	β	1	0	0	0	0	β	0	0	0	0	0		η_2
CHHD42	0	β	1	0	0	0	0	β	0	0	0	0		η_3
CHSP18	0	0	0	1	0	0	0	0	0	0	0	0		η_4
CHSP30	0	0	0	β	1	0	β	0	0	0	0	0		η_5
CHSP42	0	0	0	0	β	1	0	β	0	0	0	0	$\cdot$	η_6
WT24	β	0	0	β	0	0	1	0	0	0	0	0		η_7
WT36	0	β	0	0	β	0	β	1	0	0	0	0		η_8
WT48	0	0	β	0	0	β	0	β	1	0	0	0		η_9
HT24	β	0	0	β	0	0	0	0	0	1	0	0		η_{10}
HT36	0	β	0	0	β	0	0	0	0	β	1	0		η_{11}
HT48	0	0	β	0	0	β	0	0	0	0	β	1		η_{12}

=

WT12	HT12	MAATT18	MAATT30	MAATT42	CHDIAR18	CHDIAR30	CHDIAR42	MORBOTH18	MORBOTH30	MORBOTH42	LACT18	FMSZO	SEX	ZMARD	ZPARD	MODVOC	CONSUMP	PASTAT	ZMAOCC	MAHT	PAHT	TREAT
γ	0	0	0	0	γ	0	0	γ	0	0	γ	γ	γ	γ	γ	γ	γ	γ	γ	0	0	0
0	0	0	0	0	0	γ	0	0	γ	0	0	γ	γ	γ	γ	γ	γ	γ	γ	0	0	0
0	0	0	0	0	0	0	γ	0	0	γ	0	γ	γ	γ	γ	γ	γ	γ	γ	0	0	0
γ	0	γ	0	0	γ	0	0	γ	0	0	γ	0	γ	γ	γ	γ	0	0	0	0	0	γ
0	0	0	γ	0	0	γ	0	0	γ	0	0	0	γ	γ	γ	γ	0	0	0	0	0	γ
0	0	0	0	γ	0	0	γ	0	0	γ	0	0	γ	γ	γ	γ	0	0	0	0	0	γ
γ	0	0	0	0	γ	0	0	γ	0	0	γ	0	γ	0	0	0	0	0	0	γ	γ	0
0	0	0	0	0	0	γ	0	0	γ	0	0	0	γ	0	0	0	0	0	0	γ	γ	0
0	0	0	0	0	0	0	γ	0	0	γ	0	0	γ	0	0	0	0	0	0	γ	γ	0
0	γ	0	0	0	γ	0	0	γ	0	0	γ	0	γ	0	0	0	0	0	0	γ	γ	0
0	0	0	0	0	0	γ	0	0	γ	0	0	0	γ	0	0	0	0	0	0	γ	γ	0
0	0	0	0	0	0	0	γ	0	0	γ	0	0	γ	0	0	0	0	0	0	γ	γ	0

$$\cdot \begin{bmatrix} \xi_1 \\ \xi_2 \\ \xi_3 \\ \xi_4 \\ \xi_5 \\ \xi_6 \\ \xi_7 \\ \xi_8 \\ \xi_9 \\ \xi_{10} \\ \xi_{11} \\ \xi_{12} \\ \xi_{13} \\ \xi_{14} \\ \xi_{15} \\ \xi_{16} \\ \xi_{17} \\ \xi_{18} \\ \xi_{19} \\ \xi_{20} \\ \xi_{21} \\ \xi_{22} \\ \xi_{23} \end{bmatrix} + \begin{bmatrix} \zeta_1 \\ \zeta_2 \\ \zeta_3 \\ \zeta_4 \\ \zeta_5 \\ \zeta_6 \\ \zeta_7 \\ \zeta_8 \\ \zeta_9 \\ \zeta_{10} \\ \zeta_{11} \\ \zeta_{12} \end{bmatrix}$$

Figure 3-10 Home Diet, Supplement, and Physical Growth: Structural Equation (coefficient subscripts omitted)

Moreover, it is especially important to allow for, and estimate, errors in measurement of home diets. This is known to be substantial, as discussed above; to neglect these errors could seriously bias estimates of coefficients. While the measures of anthropometry and supplementation are not expected to show appreciable error, the full model does allow for possible errors of measurement as well as for unexplained variance in each of the 12 joint endogenous variables.

This type of model—which includes both structural equations that relate latent ("true") variables, and measurement equations relating the latent variables to observed variables that are fallible—is discussed succinctly in Jöreskog and Sörbom (1979, pp. 106–113). The computer program, LISREL,* by Jöreskog and Sörbom (1976) has been used to estimate each of the models discussed in this chapter. The program provides full-information, maximum-likelihood estimates of the parameters of sets of simultaneous equations using an iterative Fletcher-Powell (1963) algorithm for minimization.

In order to identify errors of measurement separately from errors in the equations, some constraints must be imposed on the parameters. A reasonable supposition is that the errors of measurement in each sequence are an equal proportion of the variance of the variable at that age.† A preliminary model with variables in standardized form (that is, a correlation matrix) was solved to estimate these error terms.‡ The maximum-likelihood estimates of error variances were 23 percent for home diet, 3 percent for weight, and 0 percent for the measurements of supplementation and of height. Given our prior knowledge of how measurements were made in the field, these estimates fit our expectations. The critical estimate of 23 percent error for home diets also is consistent with the correlations ranging from 0.5 to 0.6 between measures of home diets at successive ages.

Missing Data. In estimating the final form of this model (and the three others discussed later in this chapter), the covariance matrices have been generated by pairwise deletion of missing data. That is, each covariance is based upon all instances for which measures are

---

* A CDC6400 version of LISREL III, slightly modified so as to constrain variances to be nonnegative, is the computer program used throughout.

† Since the variance of each variable increases with child's age, assuming constant error variance would imply increasing reliability with age. Assuming a constant proportion, as we have done, implies a constant reliability of measurement.

‡ See Benson, *et al.* (1980, pp. 103–108) for an exact specification of this model, which slightly differs from that presented here.

available for the pair of variables—even though measures of other variables might be missing for that particular case. This procedure maximizes the use of available data and is consonant with the maximum-likelihood philosophy of making the best possible estimates of the relevant population values. Casewise deletion, while generating internally consistent Gramian matrices, discards data (for this model it would mean keeping only 243 cases out of 512 as compared to the average of 444 cases) and introduces additional sub-sampling bias (Kim and Curry, 1977).

Correlates of Diet. Maximum-likelihood solutions for the structural coefficients of this model are shown in Tables 3-1 and 3-2. Our main purpose in generating this model was heuristic: to compare the effects on growth of home diet and supplementation. Before proceeding to this comparison, we present policy-relevant correlates of children's diets in the first of these tables.

From year to year the stabilities of both home diet and supplementation are high. (These coefficients appear in the row labeled "lagged dependent" in the table; they correspond to the vertical arrows of the path diagram, Figure 3-9.) Children who eat more in one year are apt also to eat more the next. Beyond these stabilities, the two variables that account for most of the variation among children in the amount of supplement consumed are: residence in the Atole villages (TREAT); and frequency with which mothers attended supplementation centers. Differences between consumption in Atole and Fresco villages were anticipated in the description of children's diets (Figures 3-2 and 3-3). While children were free to attend the centers alone, strong association with mothers' attendance is to be expected for the youngest, and a declining association as the children get older.

Children who were still nursing during their second year (at 18 months) ate less at home and supplemented less than those who had been weaned. In Fresco villages, where the supplement was perceived as mere refreshment, mothers nursed longer; infants consumed only negligible amounts of Fresco.

Home diets of children in the villages vary significantly with cultural characteristics of their families; children with literate parents, for example, are fed more accurately. The scale labeled "MODVOC," representing the vocabulary and modernity of mothers,* has

---

* This is a principal component scale, including not only the Smith-Inkeles O-M scale and a vocabulary scale, but also aspects of child care. See the variables MODREV, PTVOC, TEACH, MAINV, and PAINV in the glossary of acronyms.

Table 3-1 Home Diet, Supplement, and Physical Growth—Structural Coefficients: Equations for Home Diet and Supplement

$\chi^2 = 511.66$; $df = 499$; $\chi^2/df = 1.03$; $P = .34$ (Number of cases: minimum = 317; average = 444: maximum = 512)

	Home Diet			Supplement		
Dependent Variable:	*CCHD18*	*CHHD30*	*CHHD42*	*CHSP18*	*CHSP30*	*CHSP42*
Mean	608.2	854.5	977.4	68.8	92.9	100.6
Standard Deviation	242.6	265.3	302.6	88.8	106.5	109.5
Structural Coefficients:						
Lagged Dependent	...	.61**	.76**	...	.71**	.86**
Home Diet	...	...	...	...	...	...
Supplement	0.	...	...	...	...	...
Weight	...	15.73	15.37	0.	0.	0.
Mother's Attendance	...	...	...	134.72**	80.30**	39.50**
Diarrhea	−122.31	−207.95	0.	0.	0.	0.
Other Morbidity	69.10	−102.50**	0.	0.	0.	−10.06
Lactation (18 mo.)	−87.09**	...	...	−13.29*	...	...
Family Size (birth)	0.	−5.42	9.63	...	...	...
Sex (male)	37.32	51.53*	0.	9.93	0.	0.
ZMARD	0.	0.	0.	0.	−7.01*	−4.85
ZPARD	29.17**	0.	13.51	4.19	0.	0.
MODVOC	42.40**	34.47**	16.04	5.72	−3.50	2.76
CONSUMP	0.	−28.48*	0.	...	...	...
PASTAT	0.	−15.31	−28.48*	...	...	...
ZMAOCC	25.34*	24.99*	13.70	...	...	...
MAHT	...	...	...	...	...	...
PAHT	...	...	...	...	...	...
TREAT (Atole)	...	...	...	102.59**	33.42**	0.
$R^2 = 1 - \psi$	.15	.49	.53	.54	.70	.76

** Coefficient greater than twice its standard error, assuming the minimum number of cases (317).
* Coefficient greater than twice its standard error, assuming the average number of cases (444).
0 Coefficient less than its standard error, assuming the maximum number of cases (512).
... Coefficient not in structural equation (value fixed at 0).

Table 3-2 Home Diet, Supplement, and Physical Growth—Structural Coefficients: Equations for Growth in Weight and Height

$\chi^2 = 511.66$; $df = 499$; $\chi^2/df = 1.03$; $P = .34$ (Number of cases: minimum = 317; average = 444; maximum = 512)

	Weight			Height		
Dependent Variable:	WT24	WT36	WT48	HT24	HT36	HT48
Mean	9.7	11.8	13.5	77.3	85.5	92.9
Standard Deviation	1.2	1.4	1.5	3.6	4.1	4.2
Structural Coefficients:						
Lagged Dependent	.77**	.94**	.96**	.93**	.96**	.96**
Home Diet	.0003*	.0003*	0.	.0009	.0012**	.0011**
Supplement	.0026**	.0015**	0.	.0054**	.0059**	.0013*
Weight	...	...	...	...	...	...
Mother's Attendance						
Diarrhea	−.68*	−.74	0.	−1.83*	−3.43**	−3.17**
Other Morbidity	0.	0.	−.21	0.	0.	.21
Lactation (18 mo.)	0.	...	...	.76**	...	...
Family Size (birth)	...	...	...	...	...	...
SEX (male)	.13	.10	0.	−.28	0.	−.24
ZMARD	...	...	...	...	...	...
ZPARD	...	...	...	...	...	...
MODVOC	...	...	...	...	...	...
CONSUMP	...	...	...	...	...	...
PASTAT	...	...	...	...	...	...
ZMAOCC	...	...	...	...	...	...
MAHT	.02**	0.	.01**	.06**	.03	0.
PAHT	.01	.01*	0.	0.	.05**	0.
TREAT (Atole)	...	...	...	...	...	...
$R^2 = 1 - \psi$	.68	.79	.86	.74	.85	.91

** Coefficient greater than twice its standard error, assuming the minimum number of cases (317).

* Coefficient greater than twice its standard error, assuming the average number of cases (444).

0 Coefficient less than twice its standard error, assuming the maximum number of cases (512).

... Coefficient not in structural equation (value fixed at 0).

the strongest effect upon the adequacy of children's home diets. Fathers' literacy (ZPARD) has a significant, but smaller, independent favorable effect.

When holding cultural characteristics of families constant, socioeconomic variables (for example, CONSUMP)* do not show strong residual effects on home diet. Material affluence, positively correlated with home diet, also is associated with the cultural characteristics that interpret the association. Children living in better homes do eat better because they are more likely to have literate parents who are more involved with their care.

Effects on Growth. Table 3-2 lists the values of the estimates of coefficients for growth. The stabilities (again labeled "lagged dependent") here account for most of the explained variance in size at each age level—an increasing proportion of variance as the children grow older. After the second year children's relative position in their group changes very little.

Our central interest in this table lies in the comparison between effects upon growth of home diet and supplementation. It is clear that variations in the consumption of supplement (mainly Atole during the second and third years of life) has an effect many times as large as variations in children's home diets. During the child's second year, for example, the estimate of 0.0054 cm growth in height per kcal per day of supplement is six times as large as the 0.0009 cm growth per kcal per day from home diet.

The large effect of increments of Atole supplementation for children eating the same home diet—contrasted with the small effect of increment in home diet for children consuming the same amount of supplement—is not consistent with the hypothesis that the total caloric value of the supplement (utilizing protein as a source of energy) is what accounts for the gains of children in Atole villages. The large effect of the supplement does suggest that increments in protein derived from Atole supplementation, although higher than currently recognized needs, are of direct value in promoting growth.† In the next section we will examine this hypothesis more directly.

---

* CONSUMP, also a principal component factor scale, includes 17 variables characterizing the family's house and possessions. See the variables HSTYP, HOUSER, WALLS, HOUSE, ROOMS, ROOF, and COOKPL in the glossary of acronyms for variables having the highest loadings on this factor.

† The assumption of even larger unreliability of measurement of home diets does not qualitatively change this comparison.

We should also note in Table 3-2 (although this will be reiterated in the next section) the positive effect of mother's lactation, consistently negative effects of incidence of diarrhea, and the relatively small effects of variations in parental stature (MAHT and PAHT) upon children's growth in both weight and height.

Calories, Protein, and Growth

To examine more directly the hypothesis we propose—that variations in protein have a direct effect on growth—we revise the

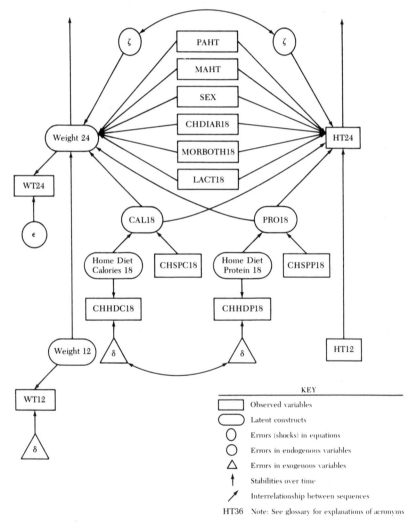

Figure 3-11 Calories, Protein, and Physical Growth: Portion of Path Diagram.

model above, replacing "home diet" and "supplement" with protein (measured in kcal units) and calories (excluding the caloric value of protein).

Revised Model of Diet and Growth. Since (in the previous model) family characteristics were presumed to affect growth through their effects upon a child's diet indirectly, but not directly, here we simplify the model, taking weight and height to be endogenous variables, and the components of diet to be exogenous. Other factors directly affecting growth in the previous model—sex, diarrhea, other morbidity, parents' heights, and mothers' lactation—again are included.

The first cycle of this model is shown as a path diagram in Figure 3-11. The same cycle sketched there is repeated for weight and height at ages 36 and 48 months, showing increments of the exogenous variables by numeric suffixes to 30 and 42, respectively. Except for replacing home diet and supplement by calories and protein, this model is like the previous one (in the right half of Figure 3-9), and in the estimates shown in Table 3-2.

Error Terms. Errors in measurement of home diet data (both calories and protein) are set at 23 percent of their variance from the earlier estimate; errors in measurement of weight are set at 3 percent. An additional correlation, between errors of measurement of components of home diet, has been introduced—represented in the path diagram by the double-headed curved arrow appearing between error terms for CHHDC and CHHDP (child's home diet calories and protein, respectively). Since the reporting by mothers of unusually large or small quantities of food consumed on the sampled days would inflate or deflate estimates of protein and caloric content proportionately, this correlation between errors was set at 0.8, approximately the same as the overall correlation between protein and calories in the home diet.*

Effects of Protein. Table 3-3 displays estimates of the structural coefficients in this model. There are no substantive differences between this solution and the previous (Table 3-2) except for the way in which children's diets have been reaggregated. The variance explained for each endogenous variable (indicated by R^2 in the bottom row)—stabilities, negative effects of diarrhea, positive effects of

---

* The magnitude of the correlation between errors of measurement is not identifiable in this model. However, the structural coefficients are robust over a range of feasible assumptions. When these correlations are set to zero there is no qualitatively important difference. The overall fit of the model, indicated by the value of χ^2, is improved by assuming a positive correlation.

Table 3-3 Calories, Protein, and Physical Growth—Structural Coefficients

$\chi^2 = 320.30$; $df = 406$; $\chi^2/df = .79$; $P = 1.00$ (Number of cases: minimum = 317; average = 437; maximum = 512)

	Weight			Height		
Dependent Variable:	WT24	WT36	WT48	HT24	HT36	HT48
Mean	9.7	11.8	13.5	77.3	85.5	92.9
Standard Deviation	1.2	1.4	1.5	3.6	4.1	4.2
Structural Coefficients:						
Lagged Dependent	.79**	.94**	.95**	.94**	.97**	.96**
Calories	0.	0.	-.0002	0.	0.	.0011
Protein	.0070**	.0056**	.0023**	.0132**	.0146**	0.
Diarrhea	-.60	-.64	0.	-1.71	-3.14**	-3.17**
Other Morbidity	.14	0.	-.24	.45	0.	.22
Lactation (18 mo.)	.10	...	...	.82**	...	...
SEX (male)	.12	.10	.06	-.30	0.	-.24
MAHT	.02**	0.	.02**	.05**	.03	0.
PAHT	0.	.01	0.	0.	.04**	0.
$R^2 = 1 - \psi$	.67	.79	.86	.74	.84	.91

** Coefficient greater than twice its standard error, assuming the minimum number of cases (317).

* Coefficient greater than twice its standard error, assuming the average number of cases (437).

0 Coefficient less than its standard error assuming the maximum number of cases (512).

... Coefficient not in structural equation (value fixed at 0).

lactation—remains as before. The model is a substantially better fit to the data than was the previous model as indicated by a value of χ^2 less than the number of degrees of freedom, and the probability of 1.00 (that, given the specifications, a random covariance matrix would not provide as good a fit).

But the model clearly does underscore the importance of protein for growth—especially during the second and third year. For children of the same height at 12 months, and consuming the same number of calories (net of protein) during their second year, an increment of 100 kcal (25 gr) of protein in their diets per day leads to 0.7 kg growth in weight and 1.32 cm growth in stature.* Given the same quantity of protein in their daily diets, however, variations in calories (net of protein) in the ranges of available food do not lead to growth in either weight or height. With constant protein intake, variations in caloric consumption must lead to variations in energy expenditure (rather than accumulation of fat) among these generally undernourished children.

Reduced Form. The reduced form of these structural coefficients, tallied in Table 3-4, is of interest for estimating continuing effects of early intervention. For example, in the row labeled PRO18 (kcal protein per day at 18 months) we see, as before, that early intervention affects growth in height during the second year by 0.0132 cm. Because of the stability—the cumulative pattern—of growth, children who enjoyed this increment during their second year, but were reduced to the population average during the third year, would still be 0.0128 cm taller at 36 months and 0.0123 cm taller at 48 months. If this one kcal/day advantage were sustained for all three years, the increment would be 0.0123+0.0140+0.0010=0.0273 cm.

Three factors that substantially impact growth and are potentially modifiable are protein consumption, incidence of diarrhea, and duration of mothers' lactation. The value of continued nursing, indicated here only as a yes-or-no categorical variable, varies with the nutritional status of the mother; our data indicate an average beneficial effect.

Unanticipated Treatment Effects. We expect some degree of

---

* Increasing the assumed error of measurement of home diets from 23 percent (derived from the previous model) to 40 percent slightly diminishes the magnitude of these estimates, yet they remain significantly positive. Given the stability of home diet (Table 3-1), it does not seem plausible for these errors to be greater than 40 percent.

Table 3-4 Calories, Protein, and Physical Growth—Reduced Form Coefficients

Dependent Variable	Weight			Height		
	WT24	WT36	WT48	HT24	HT36	HT48
Lagged Dependent:						
WT12	.7896**	.7435	.7056	0.	0.	0.
HT12	0.	0.	0.	.9401**	.9109	.8747
Calories:						
CAL18	-.0001	-.0001	-.0001	.0000	.0000	.0000
CAL30	0.	-.0002	-.0002	0.	.0004	.0003
CAL42	0.	0.	-.0002	0.	0.	.0011
Protein:						
PRO18	.0070**	.0066	.0062	.0132**	.0128	.0123
PRO30	0.	.0056**	.0053	0.	.0146**	.0140
PRO42	0.	0.	.0023**	0.	0.	.0010
Diarrhea:						
CHDIAR18	-.6034	-.5682	-.5392	-1.7123	-1.6591	-1.5931
CHDIAR30	0.	-.6389	-.6062	0.	-3.1430**	-3.0179
CHDIAR42	0.	0.	-.2872	0.	0.	-3.1664**
Other Morbidity:						
MORBOTH18	.1397	.1315	.1248	.4482	.4343	.4170
MORBOTH30	0.	.1065	.1010	0.	.0688	.0661
MORBOTH42	0.	0.	-.2401	0.	0.	.2177
Lactation:						
LACT18	.0978	.0921	.0874	.8155**	.7902	.7587
Sex (male):						
SEX	.1205	.2124	.2616	-.2969	-.2304	-.4570
Parents' Height:						
MAHT	.0158**	.0197	.0340**	.0546**	.0818	.0874
PAHT	.0032	.0139	.0117	.0094	.0504**	.0520

** Coefficient greater than twice its standard error, assuming the minimum number of cases (317).

replacement of home diet by the kind of supplement offered in the INCAP experiment. Because of the high-protein content of Atole and the effects of this increment for children's growth, even total replacement would have resulted in gains.

The availability of this "free good"—the nutritious Atole supplement—seems to have had two additional, unforeseen consequences. One is the earlier weaning of children in Atole villages, though continued nursing would have been beneficial; the other is a significant sex by treatment interaction.

If one looks closely at the difference between boys and girls—in the gap between Atole and Fresco village growth curves (comparing Figures 3-4 with 3-6, and 3-5 with 3-7)—one may detect that the advantage of Atole is systematically larger for girls than for boys. A series of cross-sectional two-way analyses of variance of weight and height by treatment and sex at different ages show highly significant interaction effects.

The differences in size between boys and girls for a number of age levels are shown in Table 3-5. In Atole villages the gap in stature narrows as children get older; in Fresco villages the gap in weight widens. By 48 months the gap between boys and girls in Atole villages is less than half the gap found in Fresco villages.

The competition for food is attenuated in the presence of this free good. While, on the average, boys eat more than girls in both Atole and Fresco villages, discrepancies in home diets during early years are smaller in Atole villages. Between families, the poorer, and within families, the less powerful, are those who benefit from the greater availability of food.

Table 3-5 Differences Between Boys and Girls in Height and Weight by Treatment and Age

	Boys' Mean Height Minus Girls' Mean Height in Centimeters		Boys' Mean Weight Minus Girls' Mean Weight in Kilograms	
Age	Atole	Fresco	Atole	Fresco
6 months	1.83	1.44	.46	.38
12 months	1.60	1.34	.40	.47
24 months	1.10	1.40	.35	.69
36 months	.71	2.15	.45	.83
48 months	.63	1.88	.41	.87

Growth and Performance

Verbal Development

The INCAP study originally focused on the effect that supplementation—alleviation of calorie/protein deficiency—might have upon child development. Particular attention was paid to cognitive development. Because of this interest, a comprehensive and eclectic battery of developmental and psychometric scales was periodically administered to children in the villages. Members of the INCAP study team have shown significant correlations between supplementation and a number of psychometric tests—specific to certain age levels by sex—when controlling for indicators of family background.

We want to accomplish two things in this section. On one hand, we want to narrow the scope of analysis by focusing attention upon two closely related indicators of verbal development; on the other hand, we hope to extend prior analyses by explicitly taking into account the developmental character of verbal performance (using the longitudinal aspects of the data base). We shall take account of, and estimate, errors of measurement in the dependent variables (verbal tests) and include a considerably more comprehensive array of control variables which might have prior and independent effects upon verbal performance.

Model of Verbal Development. The model (Figure 3-12) is shown as a path diagram. This model combines a constrained factor-analytic model with a structural equation (regression) model. The right-hand side represents the factor-analytic model. The hypothetical true value of verbal facility at each of five age levels is represented by two fallible indicators: "naming" and "recognition" (RECOG). These tests are analogous to the widely used Peabody Picture Vocabulary, assessing the ability both to name correctly an object shown in a picture and to select a picture to go with a name.

The variance of each test is partitioned into a communality (explained by the hypothetical verbal factor) and a uniqueness (represented by the epsilons shown in circles on the diagram). This uniqueness, in turn, includes both measurement error and specificity—the systematic content tapped by one type of performance, for example, "naming," which is not captured by the other, for example, "recognition."

The model allows for correlations between the errors of two tests

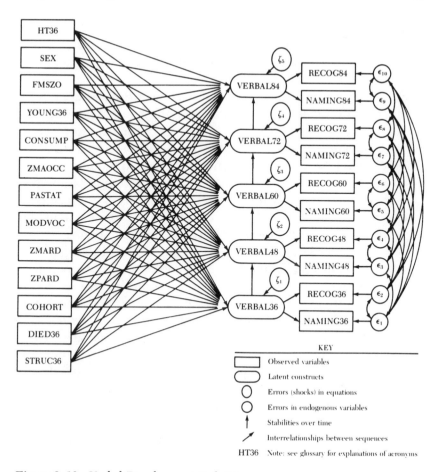

Figure 3-12 Verbal Development Path Diagram.

given on the same occasion (for example, tester effects in making consecutive assessments of related performances) as well as retest correlations between uniquenesses (for example, correlations over time between the specific aptitudes tapped by each test). These correlations are represented by the double-headed curved arrows at the extreme right edge of the diagram.

The right-hand side of the diagram represents the measurement model; the central and left-hand portions depict the simultaneous structural equation system. The vertical arrows show stabilities of verbal development—those who perform better at one age are likely to perform better at the next. This is due to the accumulation of vocabulary over time, the advantage which fluency at one point provides for subsequent language acquisition, and, possibly, to stable latent abilities that lead to individual differences. As in much prior research, we expect such stabilities to increase progressively with age.

Finally, down the left side of the diagram we have an array of independent variables that plausibly may affect verbal performance either directly, as for instance, by education or exposure, or as proxies for unmeasured factors affecting development or socialization. We take the first variable, height at age 36 months, to be a cumulative proxy for prior nutrition and absence of morbidity; this construction is in accord with our foregoing analysis. Sex is included, of course, because of the ubiquity of both earlier development and superior development (especially of verbal fluency) of females over males. The possible effect of family size upon verbal development has been the subject of antithetical hypotheses and contradictory findings. Economists, especially, favor the argument that limitation of family size reflects a more intensive investment in the socialization of the child. A large number of siblings along with members of an extended family, however, does make for a denser social environment permitting—even demanding—more verbal communication. Adults and older siblings, it is held, facilitate verbal development; younger siblings detract. Contradictory evidence in large-scale studies (Velandia, Grandon, and Page, 1978) suggests that these interpretations may be culturally dependent. Family size may not be linearly related to educative experience, or related in the same way, in different cultures.

Most of the other independent variables are more or less traditional indicators of familial advantage which, separately or collectively, may serve as proxies for the quality of the home environment. Variables with the acronyms MODVOC, ZMARD, and ZPARD have been discussed before. These three are fairly direct indicators of the richness of verbal exposure. The variable "DI-ED36" refers to the number of still-born and deceased elder siblings of the study child. This variable may serve as a proxy for some otherwise unmeasured aspects of parental care.

Again pairwise deletion has been used to generate the covariance matrix. Here the total sample was screened to eliminate children not living in the study villages at 36 months of age (dropping the former requirement that they also must have been born in the villages). This increases the maximum number of cases from 512 to 573, including children who immigrated before 36 months of age. However, because the model includes tests administered up to 84 months—and many children in the sample had not reached that age when data collection was discontinued—later tests are based on fewer cases. Age in months in 1977 (COHORT) is included as a variable to detect and control for differences between earlier and later-born children.

Because the dependent variables—the hypothetical verbal factors—are estimated in arbitrary units (scaled to the communalities of the naming test), all variables have been standardized. A correlation rather than covariance matrix is analyzed; standardized rather than raw coefficients are reported.

Coefficient Estimates. Estimates of the structural relationships for this model are shown as normalized, partial regression coefficients in Table 3-6. The strongest relationships, as would be expected, are the lagged values of the verbal factors, referred to above as "stabilities." As anticipated, these coefficients increase with age.

The most important substantive result lies in the large and highly significant predictive effect of height at 36 months on verbal performance, even when allowing for the concomitant and somewhat confounded effects of a large number of background variables. Not only does height (which we take to be a proxy for cumulative health from conception to 36 months) affect performance at age three, but also height predicts growth—learning—year by year, through age seven.

We are using height-by-age as a proxy for cumulative prior nutrition and absence of morbidity. We do not presume the linkage between height and verbal development to be direct or proximate; rather, that healthier children—more exploratory, active, and expressive—elicit a more favorable and responsive social environment (cf. Chavez, Martinez, and Yashine, 1975). The associations reported here do not distinguish between possible direct physiological effects upon capacity to learn, and indirect effects resulting from modified social environments. While theoretically it is important to sort out and specify these paths, the fact that early growth affects verbal development also is important from a policy point of view. (The extent to which height, per se, among equally healthy children, may generate positive social responses could inflate these coefficients. But we have seen in this undernourished population that heredity appears to account for little of the variation in children's height.)

Table 3-6 Verbal Development—Standardized Structural Coefficients

$\chi^2 = 42.78$; $df = 166$; $\chi^2/df = .26$; $P = 1.00$ (Number of cases: minimum = 105; average = 385; maximum = 573)

Dependent Variable:	VERBAL36	VERBAL48	VERBAL60	VERBAL72	VERBAL84
Standard Deviation	3.41	4.22	4.61	4.30	3.91
Structural Coefficients:					
Lagged dependent	...	.80**	.83**	.87**	.85**
HT36	.35**	.14*	.08*	.04	.13**
SEX	-.18*	-.07	.04	-.09*	.02
FMSZO	.09	.06	.06	0.	.15**
YOUNG36	-.06	.06	-.13	.07	.03
CONSUMP	.24**	-.08	.07	0.	.06*
ZMAOCC	0.	0.	-.05	.04	-.05*
PASTAT	-.12*	0.	0.	0.	-.10**
MODVOC	0.	0.	.07	.06	.03
ZMARD	.06	.09*	0.	.06	.05*
ZPARD	.07	0.	0.	0.	.11**
COHORT	0.	0.	0.	0.	-.02
DIED36	-.06	.03	-.10*	-.05	.17**
STRUC36	0.	-.11*	0.	-.14**	-.16**
$R^2 = 1 - \psi$	.25	.74	.82	.88	1.00

** Coefficient greater than twice its standard error, assuming the minimum number of cases (105).
* Coefficient greater than twice its standard error, assuming the average number of cases (385).
0 Coefficient less than twice its standard error, assuming the maximum number of cases (573).
... Coefficient not in structural equation.

Among the remaining independent variables included in the model (primarily as controls), sex shows the usual, earlier, verbal development and continued superiority of the girls. Family size at birth is positively, though not strongly, related to verbal development. This is congruent with the instructional thesis, but not with the investment thesis (cf. Page and Grandon, 1979). Collinearities among the remaining variables make substantive interpretations of individual statistics tenuous. We find the typical zero-order correlations—ranging from 0.25 to 0.35—between, for instance, CONSUMP and the raw verbal test scores. The partial regression of 0.24 of VERBAL36 on CONSUMP is highly significant, but effects on later development are erratic and not significant. The three variables dealing with parental literacy—MODVOC, ZMARD, and ZPARD—all have positive, but low, coefficients. Because these three variables are both conceptually and empirically interrelated, if we were primarily interested in estimating their joint effect, the variables probably should be blocked together or treated as a common factor. Because here we are primarily concerned with the effects of nutrition and health, we have not tried to sort out the independent effects of these familial background variables; rather we are content to treat them as controls.

Performance in School

About half the children in this longitudinal sample who were over age seven on January 1978 had been enrolled in school. Children with superior verbal attainment before school age are most likely to enroll (Irwin *et al.*, 1980). But there are large differences among villages in the proportion of children who enroll. The social and economic factors that lead to these village differences will be discussed in Chapter 4. Here we will focus on the performance of the hundred students in the sample who completed one or more years of school and sat for the first-year final examinations in language and mathematics.

While at one time in Guatemala nationally administered objective tests were recorded each year for children enrolled in school, this practice has been modified in recent years so that the recorded scores reflect subjective teacher judgment. This means that a variety of social and psychological factors may play directly upon these assessments, independently from whatever effect such judgments may have on measured academic performance. Western educational literature abounds with accounts of the impact of docility, dress, language, and family background upon teachers' perceptions of "good students." There is also a well-documented tendency for teachers to "normalize" estimates of performance, that is, to assess performance relatively to the distribution of achievement in a class. The "good" student in one school might appear mediocre in another where average standards were higher.

Because of this relativization of grades, and possibly idiosyncratic bases of judgment used by different teachers, the model to be developed here includes "dummy" (1- or 0-valued) variables representing the different schools.

Our path model of factors affecting teacher assessments is displayed in Figure 3-13. It consists of two simultaneous equations—one predicting assessments at about 99 months of age, the second predicting verbal attainment at 84 months. Teacher assessments are indicated by both mathematics and language grades (which are intercorrelated at $r = 0.87$). Verbal attainment, as before, is indicated by the naming and recognition test scores.

A new feature of this model is that both head circumference and stature are taken as fallible indicators of a hypothetical construct, "SIZE." Diets were last recorded for ages from 72 to 84 months— some time before most children in the sample actually enrolled. Nevertheless, diet at this age is postulated as potentially affecting both verbal attainment at 84 months and performance in school later on, as assessed by the teacher, during the following year. Because of the substantial and increasing stabilities of children's diets, it seems reasonable to assume that this earlier measure can serve as an approximate proxy for diet during the school year.

Other features of this model—sources of error, hypothesized correlations between error terms, and exogenous variables—are shown in the usual fashion. Parameters for the verbal attainment factors, and the error term for home diet estimates, were assumed from results of the preceding solutions.*

Since teacher grades, as verbal tests before, are scaled in arbitrary units, a standardized solution is presented in Table 3-7.

Looking first at the determination of verbal attainment at 84

---

* The correlation between errors (uniquenesses) of the two grades is not identifiable. Once again a range of assumptions from 0.0 to 0.5 was tried. Maximum-likelihood estimates of the free parameters were robust over these alternative assumptions.

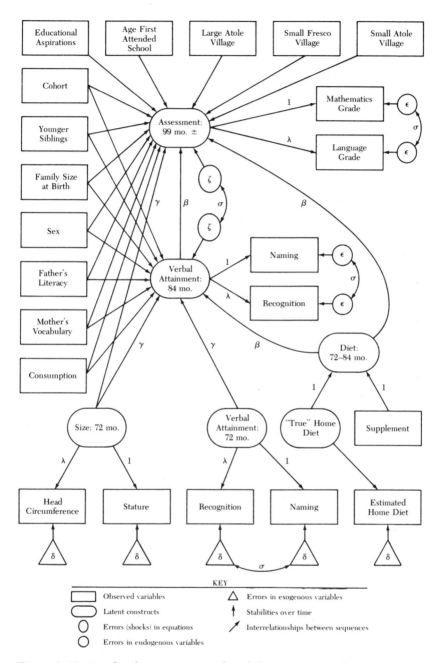

Figure 3-13 Teachers' Assessments and Verbal Attainment Path Diagram.

Table 3-7   Teachers' Assessments and Verbal Attainment—Standardized Structural Coefficients

$\chi^2 = 75.40$; $df = 186$; $\chi^2/df = .41$; $P = 1.00$ (Number of cases: minimum $= 41$; average $= 90$; maximum $= 100$)

Dependent Variable:	ASSESS99	VERBAL84
Standard Deviation	17.16	4.15
Structural Coefficients:		
VERBAL84	.40*	. . .
DIET78	.71**	.12
VERBAL72	. . .	.83**
SIZE72	0.	.30*
YOUNG72	.19	0.
FMSZO	0.	.11
ATTAGE	0.	. . .
COHORT	−.23*	0.
SEX (male)	0.	−.06
ZPARD	0.	.05
MODVOC	0.	−.06
CONSUMP	0.	−.15
EDASP	.12	. . .
VIL2 (Large Atole)	−.24	. . .
VIL3 (Small Fresco)	−.34*	. . .
VIL4 (Small Atole)	−.30*	. . .
$R^2 = 1 - \psi$	.65	.99

** Coefficient greater than twice its standard error, assuming the minimum number of cases (41).
* Coefficient greater than twice its standard error, assuming the average number of cases (90).
0 Coefficient less than its standard error, assuming the maximum number of cases (100).
. . . Coefficient not in structural equation.

months, we find again that the lagged variable (verbal attainment at 72 months) accounts for most of the variation. The coefficient is almost identical to that reported in Table 3-6. However, "SIZE" at 72 months has a considerably larger effect than that previously reported for height at age 36 months. This variable (SIZE) includes continuing effects of variations in nutrition and health between 36 and 72 months.

Turning now to factors affecting teacher assessment of performance, we see that verbal attainment has a substantial effect, as one would expect, and that there are cohort and village differences. The child's diet (total caloric value), however, is the largest and most significant factor affecting a teacher's assessment of performance, when holding constant prior verbal attainment, size, and a large number of other variables.

This clear finding* provides strong support for Latham and Cobos's (1971) thesis that current levels of energy have an important impact on learning and performance† even among children with comparable prior nutritional status and comparable levels of ability.

Summary

Rather than reiterate the text, this summary will offer a series of substantive propositions organized into two groups: (1) findings reported with confidence; and (2) findings and interpretations reported with lesser confidence.

The classification is based not only on levels of significance of individual regression coefficients but also on a combination of apparent robustness (evidenced by internal consistency across models), interpretability, and, to a lesser extent, congruence with findings in other research.

A few statistically significant coefficients which appear in this chapter are not discussed in either the text or this summary. These are primarily coefficients of social and economic indicators, included as controls but which themselves were not of central interest. Because such coefficients were included eclectically—and, to some extent, redundantly—the magnitudes of the partial regression coefficients vary from table to table and hence fail on the criterion of robustness. As indicated in various places, the focus of this chapter is primarily on the biological rather than social, backgrounds of development.

Though some of the following generalizations are stated flatly, it is to be understood that they are intended to apply to comparably undernourished populations of children, "other things being equal."

---

* In addition to the high level of significance of the individual statistic, albeit in a small sample, the model provides a very good fit overall to the data as evidenced by the value of χ^2, which is less than half the number of degrees of freedom, and the probability level of 1.00.

† Note that diet at 78 months has but slight impact on verbal growth. However, there is little room for further change in this verbal factor as measured. The value of R^2, 0.99, indicates that virtually all variance has been accounted for by age six verbal attainment and by size.

Findings Reported with Confidence

1. The availability of free high-protein supplements in the Atole villages led to:
   a. an increase in total caloric intake;
   b. partial replacement of home diet;
   c. a substantial increase in the proportion of protein in the diets of Atole village children.

2. After the introduction of supplementation, growth in weight and stature was greater in Atole than in Fresco villages.

3. Differences between Atole and Fresco villages in the growth of children in both weight and stature was greater for girls than for boys.

4. Incidence of diarrhea has a consistently negative effect upon physical growth—particularly on stature.

5. Children are more likely to consume supplement if their mothers attend the supplementation centers.

6. Stabilities of home diet, supplementation, weight, height, and verbal attainment are substantial and increase with age.

7. Boys eat more than girls, even allowing for weight differences.

8. Parental literacy is associated with the provision of better home diets.

9. Children still being nursed at 18 months were taller.

10. Increments in the proportion of protein in the diet during the second and third years of life lead to gains in weight and height.

11. Taller children perform better on verbal tests.

12. Children from more affluent homes perform better on verbal tests.

13. Girls perform better than boys on verbal tests.

14. Children with high verbal proficiency are more likely to enroll in school.

15. Children with high verbal proficiency are more likely to perform well in school.

16. Children having high current energy intakes perform better in school.

17. Parents' statures have a low correlation with children's growth.

Findings Reported with Less Confidence

18. The availability of the Atole supplement led mothers to wean children earlier.
19. Given the same consumption of protein, increments of calories (net of protein) do not lead to growth.
20. Verbal performance is enhanced by the presence of more older persons in the household.

References

BENSON, CHARLES S., SHELDON MARGEN, JUDITH B. BALDERSTON, MARIA E. FREIRE, MARI S. SIMONEN, and ALAN B. WILSON. "Education & Nutrition: Performance and Policy" Report. USAID Contract No. AID/DSPE-C-0021. April 1980 (mimeographed).

CHAVEZ, ADOLFO, CELIA MARTINEZ, and TAMARA YASCHINE. "The Importance of Nutrition and Stimuli on Child Mental and Social Development." In *Early Malnutrition and Mental Development*, edited by Joaquin Cravioto, Leif Hambraeus, and Bo Vahlquist, pp. 211–225. Uppsala, Sweden: Almqvist & Wiksell, 1974.

CHAVEZ, ADOLFO, CELIA MARTINEZ, and TAMARA YASCHINE. "Nutrition, Behavioral Development, and Mother-Child Interaction in Young Rural Children." *Federation Proceedings 34* (1975):1574–1582.

CHERNICHOVSKY, DOV, and DOUGLAS COATE. "An Economic Analysis of the Diet, Growth, and Health of Young Children in the United States." Cambridge, Mass.: National Bureau of Economic Research, Working Paper No. 146 (mimeographed), 1979.

CHRISTIANSEN, NIELS, LEA VUORI, JOSE OBDULIO MORA, and MARIA WAGNER. "Social Environment as It Relates to Malnutrition and Mental Development." In *Early Malnutrition and Mental Development*, edited by Joaquin Cravioto, Leif Hambraeus, and Bo Vahlquist, pp. 186–199. Uppsala, Sweden: Almquist & Wiksell, 1974.

CRAVIOTO, JOAQUIN, and ELSA DeLICARDIE. "Environmental Correlates of Severe Clinical Malnutrition and Language Development in Survivors from Kwashiorkor or Marasmus." In *Nutrition, the Nervous System and Behavior*, pp. 73–94. Washington, D.C.: Pan American Health Organization, 1972. ERIC ED 083 333.

CRONBACK, LEE J., and Associates. *Toward Reform of Program Evaluation*. San Francisco: Jossey-Bass, 1980.

ENGLE, PATRICIA, CHARLES YARBROUGH, JOHN TOWNSEND, ROBERT E. KLEIN, and MARK IRWIN. "Sex Differences in the Effects of Nutrition and Social Class on Mental Development in Rural Guatemala." Mimeographed, 1979.

FLETCHER, R., and M. J. D. POWELL. "A Rapidly Convergent Descent Method for Minimization." *Computer Journal 6* (1963):163–168.

IRWIN, MARC, PATRICIA L. ENGLE, CHARLES YARBROUGH, ROBERT E. KLEIN, and JOHN TOWNSEND. "The Relationship of Prior Ability and Family Characteristics to School Attendance and School Achievement in Rural Guatemala." *Child Development* 49 (June 1978):415–427.

JELLIFFE, E. F. PATRICE. *Protein-Calorie Malnutrition of Early Childhood: Two Decades of Malnutrition: A Bibliography.* Farnham Royal, Slough, England: The Commonwealth Agricultural Bureaux, 1975.

JÖRESKOG, KARL G., and DAG SÖRBOM. *LISREL III: Estimation of Linear Structural Equation Systems by Maximum Likelihood Methods: A Computer Program Manual.* Chicago: National Educational Resources, 1976.

JÖRESKOG, KARL G., and DAG SÖRBOM. *Advances in Factor Analysis and Structural Equation Models.* Cambridge, Mass.: Abt Books, 1979.

KIM, JAE-ON, and JAMES CURRY. "The Treatment of Missing Data in Multivariate Analysis." *Sociological Methods and Research* 6 (November 1977):215–240.

KLEIN, ROBERT E., JEROME KAGAN, HOWARD E. FREEMAN, CHARLES YARBROUGH, and JEAN-PIERRE HABICHT. "Is Big Smart? The Relation of Growth to Cognition." *Journal of Health and Social Behavior* 13 (September 1972):219–225.

KLEIN, ROBERT E., MARC IRWIN, PATRICIA L. ENGLE, and CHARLES YARBROUGH. "Malnutrition and Mental Development in Rural Guatemala." In *Studies in Cross-Cultural Psychology,* edited by Neil Warren, pp. 91–119. New York: Academic Press, 1977.

LATHAM, MICHAEL C., and FRANCISCO COBOS. "The Effects of Malnutrition on Intellectual Development and Learning." *American Journal of Public Health* 61 (July 1971):1307–1324.

PAGE, ELLIS B., and GARY M. GRANDON. "Family Configuration and Mental Ability: Two Theories Contrasted with U.S. Data." *American Educational Research Journal* 16 (Summer 1979):257–272.

POLLITT, ERNESTO, MITCHELL GERSOVITZ, and MARITA GARGUILO. "Educational Benefits of the United States School Feeding Program: A Critical Review of the Literature." *American Journal of Public Health* 68 (May 1978):477–481.

READ, MERRILL S. "Malnutrition, Hunger, and Behavior. 2. Hunger, School Feeding Programs, and Behavior." *Journal of the American Dietetic Association* 63 (October 1973):386–391.

READ, MERRILL S. "Nutrition, Environment, and Child Behavior." In *Nutrition and Mental Functions,* edited by George Serban, pp. 193–197. New York: Plenum Press, 1975.

RICCIUTI, HENRY. "Adverse Social and Biological Influences on Early Development." In *Ecological Factors in Human Development,* edited by Harry McGurk, pp. 158–172. New York: North-Holland, 1977.

RICHARDSON, STEPHAN A. "The Influence of Severe Malnutrition in Infancy on the Intelligence of Children at School Age: An Ecological Perspective." In *Environments as Therapy for Brain Disfunctions,* edited by Roger N. Walsh and William T. Greenough, pp. 256–275. New York: Plenum Press, 1976.

SMITH, DAVID H., and ALEX INKELES. "The OM Scale." *Sociometry* 29 (1966):353–377.

THOMSON, CAROL A., and ERNESTO POLLITT. "Effects of Severe Protein-Calorie Malnutrition on Behavior in Human Populations." In *Malnutrition, Behavior, and Social Organization,* edited by Lawrence S. Greene, pp. 19–37. New York: Academic Press, 1977.

U.S. Department of Health, Education, and Welfare. "Health Examination Survey Data from the National Center for Health Statistics." *Monthly Vital Statistics Report* (HRA) 76-1120, Vol. 25, No. 3, Supplement (June 22 1976).

VELANDIA, WILSON, GARY M. GRANDON, and ELLIS B. PAGE. "Family Size, Birth Order, and Intelligence in a Large South American Sample." *American Educational Research Journal* 15 (Summer 1978):399–416.

World Health Organization. *Energy and Protein Requirements.* Report of a Joint FAO/WHO Ad Hoc Expert Committee, Technical Report Series No. 522. Geneva, 1973.

Glossary of Acronyms Used in Chapter 3

Note: Numeric suffixes indicate age in months except for VIL.

ANIMALSS	Value of all animals owned
ASSESS	Teacher assessment of child's school performance: construct indicated by LANG and MATH
ATTAGE	Age child first enrolled in school
BIKE	Bicycle
CAL	Average daily consumption of calories excluding protein: construct indicated by CHHDC and CHSPC
CHDIAR	Proportion of days child had diarrhea during interval
CHHC	Child's head circumference in centimeters
CHHD	Child's total home diet in kcal units (CHHDC + CHHDP)
CHHDC	Child's home diet calories excluding protein
CHHDP	Child's home diet protein in kcal units
CHSP	Child's total supplement in kcal units (CHSPC + CHSPP)
CHSPC	Child's supplement calories excluding protein
CHSPP	Child's supplement protein in kcal units
COHORT	Age of child in months on March 31, 1977
CONSUMP	Housing, possessions, and salary: principal component factor scale
COOKPL	Location of cooking place: kitchen, separate, bedroom, or none
COOKTP	Type of cooking place: stone, high formal, low formal, high informal, floor, none

DIED	Number of child's siblings who have died
DIET	Child's total diet in kcal units (CHHD+CHSP)
DRAIN	Water drainage: hole in ground, floor
EDASP	Mother's educational aspirations for child
FLOOR	Floor material: blocks, cement, adobe, dirt
FMSZ	Number of persons in family
HOUSE	INCAP 1974 house scale
HOUSER	INCAP 1974 raw house scale
HSOWN	Ownership of home
HSTYP	Type of house: formal, semi-formal, rancho, improvised
HT	Child's height in centimeters
LACT	Whether mother was lactating (dummy 1- or 0-valued)
LANDAN	Land owned by family
LANG	Grade given to child by teacher in language
MAATT	Proportion of days mother attended supplementation center
MAHT	Mother's height in centimeters
MAINV	Mother's involvement in child rearing
MAOCCA	Mother's current occupation
MAOCCB	Mother's usual occupation
MAREAD	Literacy of mother
MASCH	Years of schooling of mother
MATH	Grade given to child by teacher in mathematics
MODREV	Modernity scale—modification of Smith–Inkeles O–M scale
MODVOC	Mother's modernity, vocabulary, parental involvement with child: principal component factor scale
MORBOTH	Proportion of days child had some morbidity—other than diarrhea—during the interval
NAMING	Naming psychometric test score
PAHT	Father's height in centimeters
PAINV	Father's involvement in child rearing
PAOCCA	Father's current occupation
PAOCCB	Father's usual occupation
PAREAD	Literacy of father
PASCH	Years of schooling of father
PASTAT	Father's occupation, ownership of land and animals

PLANTY   Value of land planted
PRO   Average daily consumption of protein in kcal units:
                  construct indicated by CHHDP and CHSPP
PTVOC   Vocabulary of mother
RADIO   Radio
RECOG   Recognition psychometric test score
RECORD   Record player
ROOF   Roof material: metal, tile, straw
ROOMS   Number of rooms in house
SALALL   Salaries earned by all family members
SANIT   Sanitation: septic, latrine, none
SEWING   Sewing machine
SEX   Sex (male scored 1; female scored 0)
SIZE   Physical size: construct indicated by CHHC and
                  HT
STRUC   Family structure: nuclear vs. all other
TEACH   Instruction of child by parents
TREAT   Village pair in which child lives: Atole vs. Fresco
VERBAL   Verbal attainment: construct indicated by NAM-
                  ING and RECOG
VGRA   Value of five major crops
VIL2   Larger Atole village
VIL3   Smaller Fresco village
VIL4   Smaller Atole village
WALLS   Wall material: stucco, adobe, bamboo, reed
WATER   Water source: water system, own well, public well,
                  river, or lake
WT   Child's weight in kilograms
YOUNG   Number of younger siblings
ZMAOCC   Mother's occupation
ZMARD   Mother's literacy and schooling
ZPARD   Father's literacy and schooling

Chapter 4

DETERMINANTS OF CHILDREN'S SCHOOL PARTICIPATION

by Judith B. Balderston

This chapter describes a study designed to test for the effects upon children's school participation of their prior nutrition and health conditions as well as of their parent's occupation, education, and affluence. Such analysis must take into account that, even though schooling is compulsory in Guatemala, customarily only about half the children in rural areas actually attend school, even at the lowest primary levels. Children's work activities generally take place at home or on family agricultural plots, although it will be seen that some children earn money in paid hourly work, mostly agricultural. Many children who attend school also undertake work activities during out-of-school hours.

The central question of the Berkeley study was whether the likelihood of school enrollment and subsequent achievement depends on children's early and continuing nutrition and health. Alan Wilson's analysis (see Chapter 3) shows that nutrition and health do affect children's verbal scores and school achievement. In this chapter we assume that effects of prior nutrition and health are evident by the child's attained height at age seven and that measures of concurrent nutritional intake and morbidity are available. Here we introduce economic characteristics of the child's family to examine how these appear to affect work and school activities.

It was hypothesized that several factors would shape family decisions about whether a child would attend school: (1) the economic need for a child's work, determined by family occupation and landholdings, family size and composition (including age and sex of all members), as well as by family income; (2) in addition to these measurable economic factors, parents' attitudes toward schooling, based on their own educational experience, aspirations, and expectations for their children, and attitudes about doing without children's present help in family farm or household work; (3) the influence of the child's physical development and verbal ability at school age (affected by prior nutrition and health), on the choice of whether or not to enroll the child in school.

Whether these factors exert a positive or negative influence is hard to assess a priori. Alan Wilson's findings indicate that taller children also achieve higher levels of verbal development and appear to be more successful in school. However, healthier children—seen as more valuable for work on the family farm—may find parents less willing to dispense with their help especially for children able to carry out work and school activities concurrently. Weak, small children may be seen to be of little value for work, but also as unable to profit from education. The signs of the effects of nutritional status on school participation, therefore, cannot be determined without information about the relation between family economic needs and children's work activities.

Although poor participation, dropout, repetition, and failure make for serious wastage in many educational systems, and although we suspect that malnutrition and poor health contribute to these problems, surprisingly few studies have tried to estimate the contribution of nutrition and health to school success. In fact, many school feeding programs have been instituted without evaluating their success (see Pollitt, 1978).

Many authors recognize family-background factors as inherent in school wastage but have had to rely only on measures of socioeconomic status and income (see Alexander and Simmons, 1975; and Sharma and Sapra, 1969). Since these authors did not have information about diet and health, their results imply that health, growth, and parental background can be adequately described by income or socioeconomic status, and thus that socioeconomic status and income are determinants of school participation. We know that it is highly likely that low socioeconomic status (SES) families have poorer chances of school success, less adequate diet, and generally less stimulating social environment. But it is difficult to isolate nutritional and health components, because (a) extensive nutritional data have never been collected; and (b) in purely observational cross-sectional studies, it is hard to control for SES and thus isolate nutritional and health effects on school performance.

Recently, important work by Marcelo Selowsky (1978, 1980) presents a theoretical framework for examining relationships between early health and nutrition and later school achievement and productivity. Other work has estimated relationships between nutritional status and schooling using blood-hemoglobin levels and school achievement (Popkin and Lim-Ybanez, 1980). Shortlidge's (unpublished, no date) work on the determinants of school attendance in India, using Becker's theory of household choice, explains parental decisions on the use of children's time by including family characteristics, but not characteristics of the individual child. In the present study we shall approach two of these questions—the relationships between children's nutrition and schooling and parental decisions to enroll children balanced against the need for children's work in family economic activities.

The longitudinal study carried out by INCAP made it possible to identify determinants of height, verbal development, and school enrollment (see results of such analysis as presented by Alan Wilson in Chapter 3). The supplementation program allowed us to separate out the effects of family economic status from the child's food intake since children at low-income levels were able to obtain better nutrition than otherwise would have been available. The INCAP experiment and data collection, therefore, permitted us to analyze how attained size at age seven—as a proxy measure of prior nutritional intake and morbidity, along with current measures of health—affected school enrollment* and performance. The abundant material on family work, income, wealth, parental literacy, and perceptions about the economic utility of children (collected in 1974–1975 by RAND) allowed us to look at relationships among family economic conditions, children's work activities, and school attendance.

There were three sets of information: INCAP's longitudinal data, RAND's data on family economics and children's activities, and IN-CAP's school performance data. Unfortunately for our analysis, these three sets of data were not available for the same subjects. We had to make use of available data, therefore, by carrying out the analysis in stages, which will be described in the following sections.

---

* Here school enrollment, attendance, and participation will be used interchangeably since the data collected by INCAP defined attendance as completion of the school year as indicated by grades received. Data on enrollment and actual attendance would have been preferable but were not available for all the villages.

Framework of the Analysis

A child's participation in school can be seen as the result of a number
of factors which fall into three general categories: the family's economic conditions, the child's individual characteristics, and the parents' perceptions and decisions about allocating children's time. In a
simple model we can show how family economics, child characteristics, and parental attitudes contribute directly to the child's school
participation, while recognizing that these factors themselves are
interrelated in complex ways.

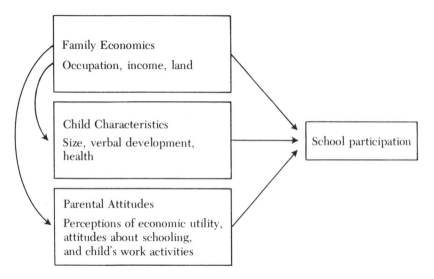

Economic conditions include family work, income, size of family,
and landholdings. Child characteristics include the child's sex, size,
health, and mental development at any age studied. Family attitudes shape the decisions that parents make, such as family size
and allocation of children's time. These attitudes control whether
parents are willing to defer children's present help in favor of
potentially higher future earnings that may result from school
attainment. Here, in order to estimate the effect on children's school
participation, we use a scale of parental perceptions of children's
economic utility, measures of parental educational aspirations for
children, and measures of the work activities undertaken by those
children.

The model above involves two kinds of simplification that must be recognized. First, family economic conditions naturally affect both the child's development and parental decisions concerning children's work; the operative mechanism, however, is not completely clear. Second, another arrow is missing that would connect the child's health and development with family attitudes about the child's work and schooling; ignoring this relationship potentially introduces bias. In a further investigation it would be important to look at the relationship of the health and size of the child and the kind of work performed, but here we had to ignore this relationship because of data limitations. In fact, we could not even estimate the full model as sketched, because data were not available that would allow us to include school, work, health, and development variables for the same group of subjects. Therefore, we had to estimate the following models separately.

Model A. The influence of economic need for the child's work was examined by way of a simple model:

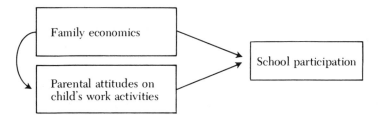

Here we looked only at economic variables—neglecting health, verbal development, and size of child because these elements were not available for that sample for which work information was available. We concentrated on how family economics appeared to affect children's work and school participation. By specifying the model in this form, we introduce bias because of the neglected variables of child's health and size which are correlated with economic group and affluence. Therefore, we tend to overestimate the effect of the need for the children's work as a cause of nonenrollment in school. We expect that in poorer families, school enrollments would be lower because of the greater need for children's economic contribution, and also because poorer families suffer from poorer nutrition and health; by omitting health and nutrition variables we tend to overstate the effect of the included variables. For this model, data were available for children born before the beginning of the nutrition experiment who were not included in the set of longitudinal data.

Model B.   Similarly, we looked at the influence of family economics, size and health, and verbal development on school enrollment. Because of the presence of the supplementation experiment
and the introduction of health care into the four communities in the
study, it was possible, partially, to separate the influence of health
and physical development from family economic background. Thus
we have another simple model:

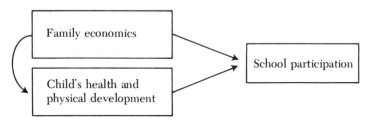

This model tends to overstate the importance of health and size by
ignoring the fact that less-affluent families may need to have their
children work more and attend school less, while more-affluent
families whose children may be better nourished and developed are
also more likely to be encouraged to attend school. Because of the
existence of the INCAP experiment, however, for the group of subjects followed since birth, it is possible that this connection has been
severed—that here family affluence is no longer a strong determinant of the children's physical growth.

Model C.   To avoid the problems inherent in Models A and B,
we sought a method that would take advantage of the two sets of data
and that would improve the power of each of the two oversimplified
models. We took the results of A (in which family economic group
appeared to relate to school enrollment) and partitioned the sample
into four economic groups: three groups of farmers and one non-
farming group. Then, returning to the three cohorts for which we
had size and health data, we used Model B to examine school-
enrollment patterns within economic groups so as to test for the
independent effects of health and size on school enrollment and
achievement. We split the sample by villages also and noted that the
differing economic characteristics of the villages produced different
patterns of school participation among villages.

Sources of Information

We had three sources of information on children's school and work activities:

1. The "R09 Files"—information collected by RAND with Rockefeller Foundation support—provided detailed measures of children's daily activities collected over four rounds, reported by mothers of 552 children, seven years of age or older in 1974–1975.
2. The INCAP schooling-information on 714 children born between 1962 and 1968 for whom there were data on school enrollment and achievement for 1972 to 1978. Material on children's paid work activities was included in these data. The information for this set of data was collected by INCAP in work supported by the National Science Foundation. Schooling data came from the Guatemalan Ministry of Education.
3. Information about school enrollment and achievement for the 543 children born between 1969 and 1971 who had been followed since birth in the INCAP longitudinal study and who were eligible to enter school by 1978.

We merged sets of files to match information by each individual child. For children born before 1969, data came chiefly from RAND files and did not include measures of growth or health. For children born between 1969 and 1971, a large set of data on anthropometry, morbidity, and diet was available in addition to information on the family from the RAND files.

R09 Files from RAND for Children Born before 1967

RAND collected information in 1974–1975 for children born before the initiation of the longitudinal study. RAND's data included measures of family work, family size, parental expectations, and an ambitious study of children's activities, from which we selected information on activities of children over age seven. A corresponding set of information was collected on the activities of children under seven, but only when the child accompanied the mother in undertaking certain activities. For children under seven, the study is more one of mothers' than of children's activities. The list of activities included chores to help the family, work for pay, farm work, etc.* The method of inquiry was to ask mothers if their children had performed such activities during the previous day. Interviews were conducted over four rounds. We selected information from the third round—considered to be more accurate than the first two rounds—which gave activities for a day when school was in session. (For detailed analysis of children's activities, see Clark 1979). Other economic information collected by RAND was merged with information on children's activities and matched by family and child. From these data we could see how children differed in activities performed according to sex, age, village, family size, and economic need.

From the list of all activities, one variable, "work," was computed to indicate whether the child undertook any work activities. Then, forming four variables, "work only," "school only," "work and school," and "neither work nor school," we performed regression and logit analysis to test hypotheses that village, family size, kind of work, and relative wealth appeared to affect the disposition of children's time. We also disaggregated by farm groups (non-farmers and subsistence, semi-subsistence, and commercial farmers) to see how children's activities appear to be related to parental economic group.

The INCAP Schooling Study for Children Born from 1962 to 1968

In a separate set of information collected by INCAP in 1978 under a study sponsored by the National Science Foundation, data were available to us to examine patterns of paid work for children of age ten to fifteen in 1978, as well as their school enrollment and achievement from 1972 to 1978. This part of the study lacked information on children's help to their families—that is, the kind of unpaid chores that were covered in the RAND activities study. Using the information so collected, in conjunction with the same set of economic variables used with the RAND data, we were able to extend the amount of information available to us about which children worked for pay and which children attended school.

---

* The complete list of activities included: prepared food for family, took care of children, went shopping, carried water, carried wood, did laundry, carried meals, did farm work, sold products, worked away from house for pay, worked within household, other activities inside house, visited relatives and other activities outside house, attended school, visited clinic, and spent nights away from house.

This set of data enabled us to look at the most recent evidence on whether children were attending school and/or had worked for pay in the past. Here, we were looking at "school," "work for pay," "school and work for pay," and "neither school nor work for pay." We carried out regression analysis, using Ordinary Least Squares, to test hypotheses that enrollment and paid work were affected by family economic activities, village, sex, and age. We aggregated, as above, all occupational groups together and then repeated the statistical tests by the four categories (non-farmers, subsistence, semi-subsistence, and commercial farmers).

Here again, as above, we had no diet, growth, or health measurements. Thus, this part of the study was useful only in showing relationships between economic variables and schooling/work patterns.

Schooling Data for Children Born from 1969 to 1971

Schooling data (collected by INCAP from Guatemalan Ministry of Education records) were available for all children who participated in the longitudinal study and who were born before December 31, 1972.

For these children a complete set of psychological, anthropometric, food intake, and morbidity variables was potentially available (and was used by Alan Wilson in his work, reported in Chapter 3). For our purposes here, selected variables included only cross-sectional data at the school-entering age, seven.

Methodology

By regression and logit analyses, we estimated determinants of school enrollments corresponding to each of the three models described previously.

Model A. School enrollment—in relation to work activities, village, age, sex, father's occupational group,* family income, mother's perception of the economic utility of children†, family size, and birth order—for children born between 1962 and 1968. Two different sets of data on work activities were used: those describing all work ac-

---

* For a full discussion of occupational groupings, see Chapter 5.

† Measures of mother's perception of economic utility of children were obtained with slight modification from the scale constructed by Mari Simonen and discussed in Chapter 6.

tivities on one day (R09 Files, round 3) and those describing only paid-work activities over a several-year period in INCAP's schooling study. School enrollment was hypothesized to be determined by the need for the child's work and parental attitudes and occupation.

Model B. School enrollment in relation to the child's developmental characteristics, for children born between 1969 and 1971. School enrollment was hypothesized to be determined by prior health and nutrition measured by height and verbal development at age seven, as well as by concurrent home diet, supplementation, health, and other variables describing family affluence, literacy, and family size. The model was also repeated excluding concurrent dietary intake.

Model C. Explanation of school enrollment by child's developmental characteristics, partitioned by village and economic groups for children born between 1969 and 1971. Here we used the same variables as in B, partitioning first by village and then by economic groups.

Findings

Model A. We considered four mutually exclusive variables: school only, work only, school and work, and neither school nor work.* In Table 4-1 we see the means and standard deviations of these variables, noting that about half of the children work and do not attend school.

We chose the variable, work, as the dependent variable and examined the influence of family economic measures on which children work.

From the regression analysis (Table 4-1) determinants of whether a child is working but not attending school appear to be: sex (girls more than boys tend to work without attending school), village (children in Village 2 are more inclined to work than those in the other villages; those in Village 4 are not likely only to work), and the child's age. R^2 results are low, indicating that there are other explanatory factors to explain the major part of the variance besides the variables included in this regression model.

Regressions were done also by occupational groups. Results

---

* We would have preferred to perform logit analyses with the four alternative activities as outcomes, but time and money constraints prevented this.

Table 4-1   Regression of Work/School Choices from RO9 (N = 515), All Villages and Occupations

Variable[a]	Mean	S.D.	Work Only Coeff.	Work Only T-Stat.
School	.0893	.2855		
Work	.4951	.5005		
School and Work	.2777	.4483		
No School	.1379	.3451		
PLBI	.5308	.3247	.1144	1.6442
PLB2	.0000	.0001	−64.6865	−.2461
COM2	.2350	.4244	.0117	.2128
COM3	.3476	.4767	−.0912	−1.8019
PERUTIL	2.5010	1.7537	.0217	1.7428
HSTYPE	2.7320	.6096	−.0596	−1.5320
SEX ($m = 1, f = 2$)	1.4913	.5004	.1366***	3.3237
Y63	.1049	.3067	−.1721*	−2.4194
Y64	.1223	.3280	−.2337***	−3.4937
Y65	.1243	.3302	−.1977**	−2.9771
Y66	.1437	.3511	−.0796	−1.2584
Y67	.1359	.3450	−.1611*	−2.4976
V2	.2796	.4492	.1266*	2.2991
V3	.1961	.3974	.0442	.6720
V4	.2175	.4129	−.3391***	−5.7887
FAMSZ	7.4893	1.6984	.0024	.1958

$$R^2 = .195$$

* p ≤ .05   ** p ≤ .01   *** p ≤ .001

[a] See Glossary on page 105 for names of variables.

showed that when we control for family economic activities, different patterns emerged by family occupational group but, because of the small sample size, there were few significant coefficients—chiefly sex, age, and village.

The schooling study carried out by INCAP in 1978 gives us the opportunity to look at school enrollment, achievement, and paid work over a several-year period in relation to the same set of economic and family variables as before. This time we break down activities into school-only, paid-work-only, school-and-paid-work, and neither-school-nor-paid-work. We concentrate on school-only, which can be seen to occur nearly half of the time. The information in this model differs from the RAND data used in the previously reported results, since it reveals several years of activity rather than a single day and does not include nonpaid work done for the family.

Table 4-2 presents regression coefficients for the analysis done for school-only as the dichotomous dependent variable. We do not show here a similar regression done for "work-and-school" as the results closely parallel these results with opposite signs. Here we see significant negative coefficients by economic groups (semi-subsistence and commercial farm groups), birth year (older children are less likely to have only attended school), and mother's expectations of child's grade attainment. Other less highly significant de-

Table 4-2 OLS Coefficients for Regression of Years of School Enrollment and Paid Work Activities of Children Born 1962–1968 (From Schooling Study)

			School Only N = 277	
Variable	Mean	S.D.	Coeff.	T. Stat.
School Only	.5379	.4995		
Paid Work Only	.0469	.2119		
School and Paid Work	.3646	.4822		
No School, No Paid Work	.0505	.2195		
PLB1	.5011	.3332	−.0739	0.7103
PLB2	.0000	.0001	−50.2894	−.1602
COM2	.2202	.4151	−.1937*	−2.4040
COM3	.3430	.4756	−.1515*	−2.0921
PERUTIL	2.4585	1.7721	−.0122	−.6933
SALALL	289.0903	451.3604	.0001	.7655
ACTGY	108.4152	261.0222	−.0001	−.4965
HSTYPE	2.7329	.6145	−.0528	−.8858
SEX (m = 1, f = 2)	1.4910	.5008	.1090	1.8186
Y63	.1264	.3328	−.3176**	−3.0435
Y64	.1444	.3521	−.2069*	−2.1027
Y65	.1444	.3521	−.1889	−1.9457
Y66	.1841	.3883	−.0719	−.7840
Y67	.2202	.4151	ne	
Y68	.1805	.3853	.0321	.3435
V2	.1552	.3628	−.1539	−1.6973
V3	.2852	.4523	−.0834	−1.0011
V4	.1697	.3760	.1250	1.3619
Family Size	7.3502	1.7867	.0203	1.2004
RWMA	.2527	.4354	.0911	1.2565
Expected Grades	5.1480	1.5095	.0647**	2.9801
RWPA	.2852	.5597	.0201	.3457
			R^2 = .172	

* p ≤ .05   ** p ≤ .01   *** p ≤ .001
ne = not entered in equation

terminants are sex (girls are more likely to attend-school-only and do nonwork-for-pay than boys) and village (Village 2 children are unlikely to attend school).

Table 4-3 gives comparisons of means and standard deviations for the same set of variables as in Table 4-2 but disaggregated by economic groups. From the breakdown of activities we see that children of all groups are equally likely to go to school at some time, and that children of semi-subsistence and commercial farmers are more likely to do paid work than are children from other occupational groups. We see also a difference in mothers' perceptions of the economic utility of children; higher perceived utility appears for children of semi-subsistence farmers, while educational aspirations are lowest for subsistence farmers. Measures of economic activity and affluence show that non-farmers and commercial farmers earn more than the other two groups. Family size of non-farmers is lower but literacy of mothers is higher.

Regressions were also done by occupational groups separately. Especially noticeable in this analysis was that children of subsistence farmers in Village 2 are most likely to do paid work. We found also that mothers' educational aspirations are clearly related to attendance in school for children of subsistence and semi-subsistence farmers. Other results from these disaggregated regressions are harder to interpret because of the small sample size and the infrequent occurrence of paid-work activities.

From the NSF-INCAP schooling study we also examined years of schooling in relation to economic and family background variables. Here, as expected, we found that children's birth year, village, mother's literacy, and educational aspirations appeared as significant determinants of the length of time spent in school.

Models B and C—School Enrollment Models for Cohorts Born 1969 to 1971. Recall that Model B related children's school participation to the child's characteristics and that Model C partitioned the groups to account for family economic activities. Based on information collected by INCAP in the longitudinal study, we examined school enrollment and achievement of children born in the first two cohorts of the nutritional experiment. These data (for children who had attained the age of seven in 1978) permitted us to hypothesize relationships between family work, parental literacy, economic factors, child's health, size, verbal fluency, sex, birth order, age, and village in relation to the child's school enrollment and achievement. In this analysis, regrettably, we had no data on children's out-of-school activities.

Table 4-3 Comparisons of Means and Standard Deviations of Variables Used in Regressions of School and Paid Work (From Schooling Study by Occupation of Father)

Variable Name	Non-Farmers (N = 43)		Subsistence Farmers (N = 99)		Semi-Subsistence Farmers (N = 61)		Commercial Farmer (N = 95)	
	Mean	S.D.	Mean	S.D.	Mean	S.D.	Mean	S.D.
School Only	.5814	.4992	.6364	.4835	.4590	.5025	.4737	.5020
Paid Work Only	.0698	.2578	.0606	.2398	.0328	.1796	.0316	.1758
School and Paid Work	.3023	.4647	.2727	.4476	.4426	.5008	.4316	.4979
No School, No Paid Work	.0465	.2131	.0303	.1723	.0656	.2496	.0632	.2445
PLB1	.2001	.3060	.5956	.3478	.5980	.3128	.4238	.2509
PLB2	.0000	.0000	.0000	.0001	.0000	.0001	.0000	.0001
PERUTIL	2.1628	1.7173	2.3131	1.8386	3.0984	1.5460	2.2947	1.7617
SALALL	453.8605	557.6657	334.0404	494.7766	159.8033	267.1866	330.7579	504.0498
ACTGY	189.4302	418.4296	62.6273	168.8538	81.3459	241.4953	123.8368	229.8465
HSTYPE	2.7442	.6580	2.6869	.5277	2.6230	.5821	2.8526	.6518
SEX (m = 1, f = 2)	1.4419	.5025	1.5051	.5025	1.4918	.5041	1.4842	.5024
Y63	.0698	.2578	.1111	.3159	.1967	.4008	.0947	.2944
Y64	.2791	.4539	.1313	.3359	.1311	.3404	.1474	.3564
Y65	.0930	.2939	.1717	.3791	.0820	.2766	.1579	.3666
Y66	.1628	.3735	.1818	.3877	.1475	.3576	.2105	.4098
Y67	.2093	.4116	.2121	.4109	.1967	.4008	.2421	.4306
Y68	.1860	.3937	.1919	.3958	.2459	.4342	.1474	.3564
V2	.0930	.2939	.1717	.3791	.1475	.3576	.1579	.3666
V3	.4186	.4992	.1717	.3791	.1148	.3214	.4632	.5013
V4	.1163	.3244	.2828	.4527	.2131	.4219	.0421	.2019
Family Size	5.5581	1.9062	7.3838	1.3455	7.7705	2.0363	7.4632	1.7370
RWMA	.3721	.4891	.1919	.3958	.2623	.4435	.2947	.4583
Educational Aspirations	5.4884	1.4699	4.8182	1.6682	5.2623	1.3404	5.2842	1.3889
RWPA	.1163	.9053	.1717	.3791	.2787	.5811	.4632	.5614

Preliminary analysis investigated relationships between child's size at seven years, concurrent health and diet, and measures of family economics. Differences between villages are apparent: In Village 2, family affluence appears to have a significant positive effect on enrollment, while amount of family economic activity has a significant negative effect. In the other villages these coefficients are not statistically significant. Village 1 shows a positive effect of home-diet protein as well as a negative effect for the proportion of older siblings in the subject's family on school enrollment.

In a stepwise regression, Table 4-4 gives results of regressing school enrollment on height, health, and family background factors. Here, from the series of related models which involve an increasing number of explanatory variables, we see how economic factors first, then parental literacy, and, finally, child-development variables appear to affect enrollment. These results provide strong evidence (controlling for economic factors and other characteristics of the family) that the child's health and his height and verbal development at age seven appear to affect school participation significantly.

Table 4-5 shows the results of regressions done by village. Since Village 2 has consistently shown low school participation and high involvement of children in the work force, our breakdown was done by Village 2 compared to Villages 1, 3, and 4 combined. Different patterns emerge to explain school enrollment. In Village 2 family affluence is the only variable to show a significant positive effect on school attendance. (This is also consistent with the results found when nutritional data were included.) For Villages 1, 3, and 4 positive determinants of enrollment are sex (boys attend more than girls), age, verbal scores, height, and father's literacy.*

We now move to Model C, which takes account of the family's need for the child's work by partitioning the sample into economic groups. Table 4-6 gives means and standard deviations for variables used in the regressions of school enrollment, divided by fathers' occupational groups. Here we see differences by family occupation in the proportion of children going to school. Non-farming families in the longitudinal sample had to be excluded because of low sample size but, for the others, Table 4-7 (giving the results of regressions) shows that patterns differ by level of economic activity and land-holdings. Again, we see that to live in Village 2 makes for a

---

* Logit analysis, performed for the same variables and groupings, were highly consistent with these findings.

Table 4-4   OLS Coefficients for Stepwise Regressions for School Enrollment (N = 184) (Levels of Significance in Parentheses)

Variable	Mean	S.D.	Step 1		Step 2		Step 3		Step 4	
Enroll	.6467	.4793								
Sex	.5217	.5009	.1508**	(.014)	.1497***	(.013)	.1562**	(.009)	.1513**	(.011)
Y69	.4837	.5011	.4478**	(.000)	.4527***	(.000)	.4494***	(.000)	.4460***	(.000)
Y70	.4347	.4971	.3890***	(.001)	.3696***	(.001)	.3738***	(.001)	.3718***	(.001)
V2	.2880	.4541	-.2893***	(.001)	-.2780**	(.002)	-.3047***	(.001)	-.3665***	(.000)
V3	.2337	.4243	.2038*	(.036)	.1811	(.059)	.1764	(.062)	.1112	(.248)
V4	.2120	.4098	-.0163	(.857)	.0174	(.847)	-.0012	(.989)	-.0334	(.706)
VCRA$	347.1641	623.4997	-.00002	(.966)	-.00002	(.977)	-.0001	(.817)	-.00001	(.880)
ORDR6	.5973	.1576	-.5311*	(.026)	-.5537*	(.019)	-.5260*	(.024)	-.4907*	(.032)
FMSZ6	6.9402	1.7561	.0155	(.454)	.0230	(.268)	.0212	(.299)	.0282	(.168)
SALALL	196.6141	299.8552	.0002	(.147)	.0002	(.103)	.0002	(.104)	-.0002	(.106)
ACTGY	67.1647	174.7513	.00001	(.958)	.00002	(.882)	-.00001	(.974)	-.0001	(.755)
PLB1	.6179	.3380	.0442	(.668)	.0717	(.487)	.0566	(.577)	.3056	(.724)
PERUTIL	2.4022	1.7806	-.0324	(.069)	-.0342	(.052)*	-.0344*	(.047)	-.0317	(.064)
CONSUMP	.0343	.9991	.1663***	(.000)	.1510***	(.000)	.1298***	(.001)	.0963*	(.018)
RWMA	.2391	.4277			.0567	(.448)	.0399	(.588)	.0388	(.594)
RWPA	.4022	.4917			.1438*	(.029)	.1450*	(.025)	.1325*	(.038)
RECOG4	33.7609	4.0065					.0195**	(.011)	.0154*	(.048)
HTC16	104.8109	4.3869							.0150*	(.043)
CHHLTH6	.6685	.3234							.1728	(.077)
			$R^2 = .359$		$R^2 = .384$		$R^2 = .407$		$R^2 = .431$	

$* \ p \leqslant .05$ $** \ p \leqslant .01$ $*** \ p \leqslant .001$

Table 4-5 OLS Coefficients for Regression of School Enrollment with Village 2 and Villages 1, 3, and 4

	Village 2 (N = 53)				Villages 1, 3, 4 (N = 131)			
Variable	Mean	S.D.	Coeff.	Level of Signif.	Mean	S.D.	Coeff.	Level of Signif.
ENROLL	.3396	.4781	—	—	.7710	.4218	—	—
SEX	.5660	.5004	.1107	(.412)	.5038	.5019	.1835**	(.005)
Y69	.4906	.5047	.4681	(.068)	.4809	.5016	.4648***	(.000)
Y70	.4151	.4975	.2515	(.330)	.4427	.4986	.4292**	(.001)
RWMA	.2075	.4094	.2248	(.195)	.2519	.4358	.0435	(.610)
RWPA	.3396	.4781	.2164	(.151)	.4275	.4966	.1590*	(.035)
VGRA$	541.3140	990.9916	−.00001	(.933)	268.6149	364.4617	.0001	(.585)
ORDR6	.6136	.1627	−.6454	(.161)	.5907	.1556	−.3280	(.232)
FMSZ6	7.0377	1.7316	.0209	(.650)	6.9008	1.7709	.0351	(.136)
SALALL	246.7358	326.7757	−.00004	(.848)	176.3359	287.0863	.0001	(.264)
ACTGY	52.4981	176.3489	−.0007	(.082)	73.0985	174.4287	.0002	(.238)
PLB1	.6409	.3246	−.2990	(.264)	.6086	.3441	.1523	(.180)
PERUTIL	3.0566	1.4730	.0007	(.990)	2.1374	1.8304	−.0315	(.086)
HTC16	106.3189	4.0927	−.0078	(.634)	104.2008	4.3691	.0255**	(.002)
CHHLTH6	.6052	.3567	.2025	(.321)	.6941	.3066	.0435	(.706)
RECOG4	34.2830	3.5701	.0004	(.985)	33.5496	4.1643	.0167*	(.049)
CONSUMP	−.2025	1.0398	.1730*	(.041)	.1301	.9698	−.0062	(.880)
			$R^2 = .493$				$R^2 = .360$	

* $p \leq .05$ ** $p \leq .01$ *** $p \leq .001$

Table 4-6 Comparisons of Means and Standard Deviations of Variables Used in Regressions of Children's School Enrollment on Size, Health, and Family Economic Variables (Children Born 1969–1971)

Variable	Non-Farmers (N = 12)		Subsistence Farmer (N = 65)		Semi-Subsistence (N = 47)		Commercial (N = 65)	
	Mean	S.D.	Mean	S.D.	Mean	S.D.	Mean	S.D.
ENROLL	.8333	.3892	.5385	.5024	.6596	.4790	.7231	.4510
SEX	.3333	.4924	.5385	.5024	.5745	.4998	.5231	.5034
Y69	.5000	.5224	.4308	.4990	.5745	.4998	.4615	.5024
Y70	.2500	.4523	.4923	.5038	.3404	.4790	.4615	.5024
V2	.1667	.3892	.2462	.4341	.3191	.4712	.3385	.4769
V3	.2500	.4523	.1846	.3910	.0851	.2821	.3846	.4903
V4	.1667	.3892	.3538	.4819	.2128	.4137	.0769	.2685
RWMA	.6667	.4924	.1692	.3779	.2766	.4522	.2462	.4341
RWPA	.5833	.5149	.2308	.4246	.4468	.5025	.5231	.5034
VGRA$	208.9806	229.5051	91.4631	75.3192	196.5499	113.1571	746.2240	916.8300
ORDR6	.7017	.1563	.5800	.1476	.5808	.1503	.6120	.1706
FMSZ6	6.5833	1.3790	6.8308	1.6160	6.8723	1.9849	7.1231	1.7545
SALALL	603.8333	507.0945	196.0769	299.1494	142.8085	176.5176	213.3692	348.3545
ACTGY	55.2000	172.0033	53.7846	157.4257	62.6723	183.2678	80.8354	182.3494
PLB1	.6063	.4482	.9608	.1519	1.000	0	.5894	.2949
PERUTIL	1.7500	1.7645	2.1077	1.8466	2.9149	1.5719	2.4154	1.7931
HTC16	106.4417	3.4516	104.1092	4.8542	104.9362	4.4806	105.2877	3.8158
CHHLTH6	.5903	.3292	.6652	.3321	.6622	.3095	.6792	.3334
NAMING4	23.7500	3.8168	19.5538	5.0468	22.7447	4.4841	21.0308	4.0349
RECOG4	35.7500	3.0488	32.6154	4.2489	34.7872	3.9379	34.0308	3.6656
CONSUMP	.9338	.9088	-.2221	.9392	-.0150	.9772	.2394	.9913

Table 4-7 OLS Coefficients for Regression of Children's School Enrollment on Family Economic and Background Variable and Size and Health by Family Occupation (Cohorts Born 1969–1971)

Variable	Subsistence Farmers		Semi-Subsistence Farmers		Commercial Farmers	
	Coeff.	Level of Signif.	Coeff.	Level of Signif.	Coeff.	Level of Signif.
SEX	.1861	(.180)	.3482**	(.010)	.1879	(.129)
Y69	.4447	(.063)	.1541	(.455)	.7118***	(.001)
Y70	.3659	(.120)	.1273	(.582)	.6152**	(.005)
V2	-.4043	(.077)	-.2714	(.118)	-.3719*	(.033)
V3	.2271	(.313)	1.1003**	(.003)	-.1084	(.544)
V4	.1233	(.487)	-.1977	(.237)	.0672	(.794)
RWMA	-.1189	(.503)	.1380	(.318)	.0057	(.964)
RWPA	.1328	(.416)	.1499	(.242)	.1498	(.196)
VGRA$	.0001	(.559)	.0001	(.831)	-.00004	(.417)
ORDR6	-.1215	(.821)	-1.3199**	(.009)	-.5306	(.279)
FMSZ6	.0347	(.463)	.0537	(.151)	.0441	(.299)
SALALL	.0003	(.198)	-.0001	(.849)	.0001	(.475)
ACTGY	.0001	(.881)	-.0003	(.429)	-.0004	(.191)
PLB1	-.5468	(.200)	not entered		-.2426	(.291)
PERUTIL	-.0560	(.099)	-.0045	(.922)	.0102	(.766)
HTC16	.0813	(.561)	.0287*	(.050)	.0065	(.717)
CHHLTH6	.2031	(.306)	-.1774	(.373)	.2100	(.236)
RECOG4	.0109	(.501)	.0401	(.026)	.0243	(.149)
CONSUMP	.0943	(.355)	.2391**	(.013)	.0323	(.638)
	$R^2 = .497$		$R^2 = .741$		$R^2 = .482$	

$* \ p \leq .05$ $** \ p \leq .01$ $*** \ p \leq .001$

significant negative influence on school enrollment, but Village 4 produces a positive influence. Among semi-subsistence farmers, the child with fewer older siblings is more likely to go to school, as is the taller, more verbal child. More affluence in families also tends to have an increased positive effect on school enrollment.

A final table, 4-8, shows the results of regressing school-achievement measures on the same set of variables as before. School achievement was measured in terms of school promotion rates, and scores in language and mathematics (as assigned by teachers at the end of the school year). Few significant explainers appear here. Factors that explained participation in school did not appear to determine school performance once the child was in attendance. Verbal development alone appears to be of positive significance in determining achievement. These results are consistent with those obtained by Alan Wilson in Chapter 3 of this book.

Summary of Results

In this chapter we have examined determinants of school participation of children in four rural villages in Guatemala. There, as in many other rural communities in the world, the child's school participation appears to be affected by parents' need for their children's help, by parents' perception of the value of schooling, and by the child's apparent competence. We have seen in this analysis that, in one village where work is readily available and where parents' educational background is relatively low, school participation is affected positively by family affluence but not by apparent differences in the child's height, health, or verbal proficiency. In the other villages, where parents have had relatively more education and work is not so readily available for children, the factors of height and verbal performance at age seven are positively and highly significantly related to school enrollment.

When family economic groups were separated, it is seen that for children of semi-subsistence farming families, decisions on enrollment appear to be positively determined by affluence of parents, size of child, and by the child's position in the family—children born earlier in the family order are more likely to attend school than those with older siblings.

We find differences in school participation by sex; schooling for girls is less frequent than for boys, and girls' work in the household

Table 4-8 Regression Results for Achievement Assuming Child Is Enrolled (N = 119)

Variable	Mean	S.D.	Promotion Rate		Average Math Score		Average Lang. Score	
			Coeff.	T-Stat.	Coeff.	T-stat.	Coeff.	T-Stat.
PROMOTION RATE	.5421	.4249	—	—	—	—	—	—
AVERAGE MATH	60.1244	17.6321	—	—	—	—	—	—
AVERAGE LANG.	60.7008	18.5801	—	—	—	—	—	—
SEX	.5630	.4981	-.1251	-1.6182	-4.0895	-1.2956	-4.8213	-1.4949
Y69	.5042	.5021	.0584	.2670	2.6058	.2925	-1.0851	-.1192
Y70	.4622	.5007	.0692	.3194	.2157	.0244	-1.3326	-.1474
V2	.1513	.3598	-.3336*	-2.5595	-12.3837*	-2.3267	-18.0132***	-3.3122
V3	.2857	.4537	-.1693	-1.3893	-5.0128	-1.0072	-5.7285	-1.1265
V4	.2353	.4260	-.2660*	-2.4660	-14.4254***	-3.2748	-8.9604*	-1.9915
RWMA	.2857	.4537	-.0603	-.6668	4.9890	1.3513	4.0111	1.0633
RWPA	.4790	.5017	-.0378	-.4507	-2.4349	-.7101	-2.6753	-.7636
VGRA$	330.3182	439.9829	.0002	1.8330	.0075	1.7974	.0091*	2.1344
ORDR6	.5838	.1630	.0539	.1666	4.4937	.3399	2.5477	.1886
FMSZ6	6.9076	1.8226	-.0461	-1.5540	-1.6038	-1.3233	-2.0784	-1.6783
SALALL	211.7563	336.6810	-.0001	-.7978	-.0020	-.3734	-.0028	-.5072
ACTGY	77.4840	181.3413	.0000	.1538	.0076	.8309	.0068	.7266
PLB1	.6063	.3499	-.0973	-.7660	3.9463	.7610	1.5253	.2879
PERUTIL	2.1597	1.8411	-.0154	-.7099	-.1231	.1390	-.0642	-.0710
HTC16	105.3008	3.9990	.0112	1.0704	.5745	1.3455	.2084	.4776
OLDSIB	.5966	.8667	-.0030	-.0466	-.6231	-.2337	.1628	.4268
CHHCTH6	.7198	.2972	.0138	.1010	-4.1278	-.7375	-5.4443	-.9520
RECOG4	34.2941	3.8628	.0268**	2.6413	1.1018**	2.6546	1.4947***	3.5246
CONSUMP	.2412	.9452	.0588	1.0148	3.1250	1.3217	3.8264	1.5839
			$R^2 = .280$		$R^2 = .303$		$R^2 = .344$	

* p ≤ .05   ** p ≤ .01   *** p ≤ .001

apparently is more valued. The perceived value of literacy for girls apparently is lower than for boys.

These findings, coming from the longitudinal nutritional experiment, make it possible to separate nutrition, health, and developmental characteristics of the child from the family's economic background. Here, when economic and family background factors are kept constant, size and health of children act as independent, positive determinants of children's school attendance and performance. These results should have significance for policy planning purposes.

References

ALEXANDER, LEIGH, and JOHN SIMMONS. *The Determinants of School Achievement in Developing Countries.* Washington, D.C.: International Bank for Reconstruction and Development, Staff Working Paper #201, March.

CLARK, CAROL. "Relation of Economic and Demographic Factors to Household Decisions Regarding Education of Children in Guatemala." Unpublished Ph.D. dissertation, University of Michigan, 1979.

POLLITT, ERNESTO, MITCHELL GERSOVITZ, MARITA GARGIULO. "Educational Benefits of the United States School Feeding Program: A Critical Review of the Literature." *American Journal of Public Health 68* (May 1978):477–481.

POPKIN, BARRY, and MARISOL LIM-YBANEZ. "Nutrition and School Achievement." *Social Science and Medicine,* forthcoming.

SELOWSKY, MARCELLO. *The Economic Dimensions of Malnutrition in Young Children.* Washington, D.C.: International Bank for Reconstruction and Development, Staff Working Paper #294, October 1978.

SELOWSKY, MARCELLO. "Nutrition, Health, and Education: The Economic Significance of Complementarities at Early Ages." Paper presented at the International Economic Association Congress, Mexico City, August 1980.

SHARMA, R. C., and C. L. SAPRA. *Wastage and Stagnation in Primary and Middle Schools in India.* New Delhi: National Council of Educational Research and Training, 1969.

SHORTLIDGE, RICHARD. "A Socioeconomic Model of School Attendance in Rural India." Unpublished paper.

Glossary of Variables Used in Chapter 4

ACTGY	Gross income from nonagricultural activities (excluding wages)
CHHLTH6	Child's health (proportion of days' healthy) at 78 months
COM2	Semi-subsistence farmer
COM3	Commercial farmer
CONSUMP	House possessions and salary, a factor score
EDASP	Mother's educational aspirations for child
ENROLL	School enrollment, no = 0, yes = 1
FAMSZ	Family size
FMSZ6	Family size at child's sixth year
HSTYPE	House type
HTC16	Height in centimeters at 72 months
ORDR6	Proportion of older siblings at 72 months
PERUTIL	Perceived economic utility of children
PLB1	Percent family labor used
PLB2	Percent family labor used standardized by value of land planted
RECOG4	Recognition, psychometric test, age 72 months
RWMA, RWPA	Mother's and father's literacy (0,1) respectively
SALALL	Total wage income accruing to household
SEX	Female = 0, male = 1, unless otherwise specified
V2, V3, V4	Villages 2, 3, and 4
VGRA$	Gross value of agricultural production
Y69, Y70	Birth year

Chapter 5

EDUCATION AND AGRICULTURAL EFFICIENCY*

by Maria E. Freire

A recurrent theme of this book has been the multiple relations that exist between education, nutrition, and various socioeconomic factors. From a methodological viewpoint, and to introduce this section, we can visualize this set of relations as part of a large three-phase loop depicting (1) how children's nutritional status is determined by a variety of socioeconomic factors and environmental conditions; (2) how children's nutrition affects school performance; and (3) how the effects of school performance can be projected into the future. The rationale of (3) is that more schooling for today's children will enhance their ability to become better farmers, earn higher incomes, and, consequently, give their own children better nutrition and more education.

Chapters 3 and 4 addressed the first two phases of this loop by studying what determines nutritional and educational status of Guatemalan children. This section takes up the third phase. Assuming that what is found true for today's farmers will remain valid for the next generation (when the children studied in earlier sections become adult farmers), we will examine whether more education for

---

* This chapter is a selective summary of findings presented elsewhere: See M. Freire, "Assessing the Role of Education in Rural Guatemala: The Case of Farm Efficiency" (Unpublished doctoral dissertation, Department of Economics, University of California–Berkeley, 1979). I would like to thank Drs. Lawrence Lau and Dean Jamison for making available to me some work not yet published. See: D.T. Jamison and L.J. Lau, *Farmer Education and Farmer Efficiency* (The Johns Hopkins University Press, Baltimore), forthcoming, and M. Lockeed, D. Jamison, and L.J. Lau, "Farmer Education and Farmer Efficiency: A Survey," in Timothy King (ed.), *Education and Income* (Washington, D.C.: The World Bank, 1980).

some present farmers has any influence on the ability to extract the maximum income from their physical and human endowments.

Framework of the Analysis

The rationale for assuming that schooling affects economic performance is that education is a vehicle for helping the farmer (or farm-manager) to gather and use the information he needs to make decisions, and to organize production both in everyday matters and at critical times—for example, when deciding to plant new crops or introduce new production techniques. Thus, for farmers who pursue the same goals—maximization of profits, maximization of food production for house consumption, etc.—one expects that those with more education are also those who are more successful in managing factors of production to attain those goals.

To test whether this argument holds among our Guatemalan farmers (described in Appendix 5–1—and, more generally, in Chapter 2—for the whole sample, and by villages) calls for some preliminary analysis with respect to three necessary assumptions: (1) farmers have the same objectives, regardless of educational level, wealth, or age; (2) farmers can choose among crops, factors of production, input combinations, and so on, depending on their information and judgment on the best way to achieve goals; and (3) farmers' decisions are not limited by socioeconomic factors that are related to the level of education of the farmer. If these three conditions are present for our Guatemalan farmers, we shall be able to analyze the effects of education on efficiency. Let us expand on this topic further.

First, farmers may have different production objectives. For example, large farmers operating for the market are more likely to aim at maximizing profits than are small farmers, producing mainly for household consumption, who try instead to maximize farm production. Farmers who have easy contact with labor and commodity markets may allocate labor resources to work-for-wages if this leads to greater household income; those with less market knowledge, however, may use relatively more of their own labor for home farming in the fear that otherwise home consumption needs will be unsatisfied.

Second, our testing will be validated only if the existing environment permits farmers to choose among alternative options of cultivation or labor allocation. It may happen, however, as emphasized by several authors (see, for example, Reynolds, 1975), that a long and historical experience has led to traditional processes of cultivation from which people have learned how to produce as much as possible from limited resources—thus reducing the variation of production processes to insignificant levels. Such farmers have little room to make different choices or use a variety of managerial skills.

Fortunately for this analysis, our villages are not typical of the completely traditional and secular peasant society. In fact, while many farmers in the study villages continue to grow traditional food staples (corn and beans) without chemical fertilizers, many others have introduced cash crops (tomato, chili, and *maicillo*—sorghum) to sell in the market, and do use cash inputs to grow both food and cash crops. Moreover, we have detected substantial differences among farmers regarding input combinations, such as the amount of labor used per acre of land planted, or the amount of cash inputs per man-day. Our sample pertains, therefore, to the group of villagers for which cross-sectional analyses have successfully shown the positive effect of education on farmers' managerial skills (see M. Lockeed, J. Jamison, and L. Lau, 1980)—examples which demonstrate how change and the effect of education are breaking into secular and traditional processes, allowing for more favorable attitudes among literate people toward innovation, as stressed by Schultz (1975). In environments subject to change, people certainly react in different ways, depending on their knowledge of new processes and capacity to acquire such knowledge. Educated farmers, to whom school has provided contact with new ideas, are more likely to accept change than less-educated peers. The effects of education on farmers' managerial skills, therefore, are identified more easily in environments where change is occurring.

Last, even if the development stage of the study villages does allow for choosing among several alternatives, other factors could act to limit choice, and thus flaw our results. For example, less-educated farmers may operate with smaller units because of having come from poorer families (in itself a possible indication of low educational level and small plots) or because of credit restraints (associated with those minimal landholdings) which limit the possibility of renting more land.

In short, the effect of farmers' education on their ability to achieve the most from their factors of production can be tested when the farmers studied pursue the same objectives and face the same type of socioeconomic constraints; otherwise, results will reflect differences in objectives and constraints rather than differences in educational level. These limitations, to be borne in mind throughout this analysis, explain why we do a preliminary analysis of our data before presenting the results of econometric testing.

This chapter has three parts. Part I presents the data and sketches a preliminary analysis to see if conditions discussed above are met, or whether farmers should be aggregated into more homogeneous groups for which the assumption of common objectives and constraints then would be likely to hold. Part II introduces our rationale for aggregating subjects into three major groups according to market participation and size of landholdings. Part III presents the testing procedure, defines the concept of farming efficiency, and discusses the results. Technical notes are provided in Appendix 5-2, adding some details which were left out of the main text for the sake of simplification.

Our analysis is carried out on the assumption that *literacy* represents the best educational variable for the sample. The fact that, on the average, farmers in the study show less than one year's schooling (and that 65 percent are illiterate) leads us to another assumption. If education explains differences in managerial efficiency between literate and illiterate farmers, we then need no further disaggregation of data on literate farmers (that is, by years of schooling). The original study, of which this is but an extract, included such further disaggregation, but the quality of results was not improved enough to justify giving up the simplicity of dividing the sample into only these two groups: literate and illiterate farmers.

Part I: Data and Preliminary Analysis

The analysis focuses on 510 family farmers in the four villages for which farm-management data were available. Data collected by the RAND-Rockefeller Guatemala Project in 1975 contain cross-sectional information for farming activities carried out during one year: 1974. Data collection was made at a single point in time (relying on the recollection of farmers answering the questionnaire) and checked by a second interview some time later.

The information is fairly complete. Data exist on farm production, both consumed and sold; cost of cash inputs and hired labor; size and value of area planted; family and hired labor (in man-days)—all of them disaggregated at the crop level. Information also includes family labor working for wages outside the family unit, average wage paid to hired labor, and earnings from working for wages.

This preliminary analysis starts with the following assumptions:

1. All farmers seek to maximize household net income (which implies maximizing farm profits and income for wages—see Technical Appendix); or to maximize household food production.

2. Farmers have a common production function; that is, the same production techniques are available to all farmers, so that the same factor combinations yield the same output per unit of factor used.

3. Markets (for goods and labor services) are competitive, allowing farmers to hire and sell labor services, use chemical fertilizers and cash inputs, and plant any mix of crops, according to personal goals and management skills. Management skills can be measured in terms of how close farmers' factor combinations are to those optimal combinations derived from standard economic conditions.

4. Land (measured in equivalent quality units) is the only fixed factor in the short run; this means that profit or production maximization can be translated into profit-per-land-unit or production-per-land-unit maximization; labor and cash inputs are variable factors where their level is chosen in such a way as to maximize the farmer's objectives.

5. Education (literacy) affects management ability in the sense that literate farmers are more able to choose that combination of inputs (labor, land, and cash inputs; or labor-land, and cash-inputs-land) and outputs (crops) that maximize their objective.

Using assumptions 2 and 4 (a common production function and land fixed in the short run) we try to gain some insights on whether farmers have the same goals (assumption 1); whether markets are competitive, or whether farmers with different education face different market constraints (assumption 2); and whether education affects management-ability/farm-efficiency (assumption 5). For the moment, we use profit-per-land-unit and yield-value-per-land unit as an index of efficiency, assuming that when land is fixed, farmers try to maximize the results obtained per unit of land cultivated.

A simple way to proceed is to analyze whether the two groups of farmers of our sample obtain different levels of profit (or production) per unit of land; if so, we will try to see whether this is so because of differences in input combinations, or whether the differences prevail even when both groups use the same combination of production factors. Table 5-1 presents some descriptive statistics.

The above figures present some consistent differences between literate and illiterate farmers. On the average, literate farmers have access to more land, both in size and in quality units. Levels of agricultural production, farm profit, and household income of literate farmers surpass those of illiterate farmers; literate farmers use slightly more labor and almost twice as much inputs. In terms of land productivity and input combinations the literate group obtains higher yields per land unit, higher profits per land unit, and higher yield per man-day; factor combinations for literate farmers show greater intensity of cash inputs and less use of labor-per-land-unit. The amount of cash-inputs per man-day is still higher. In short, *literate farmers* seem to *obtain higher levels of land and labor productivity,* as well as *higher profits per land unit, using relatively more cash inputs and fewer labor services* than their illiterate neighbors (that is, literate farmers substitute cash inputs for labor).

Are we able to conclude from this that one group of farmers has a managerial edge over another because of literacy? There are two possible answers to this question. The first is *yes*: Educated farmers have better information on factor prices and can, therefore, arrange their factor combinations in order to maximize profits per unit of land. Moreover, literate farmers may be using a better mix of outputs, for their advantage in *production* per land unit is even greater than that with respect to *profits* per land unit. The second answer is *no*: Educated farmers are not better managers, they simply are able to borrow more money because they are literate and because they own more land. Illiterate farmers, on the other hand, must substitute labor for cash. Here, it is difficult to make comparisons of the efficiency of the two groups, as they face different relative prices for their inputs.

What about objectives? Can we infer from the above values that both groups share the same production goals? Not with the above values. However, using the estimates for a Cobb-Douglas production function (which we will describe in Part III), we find that illiterate farmers have a labor marginal productivity rate that is lower than the market wage-rate and lower, as well, than the earnings that they would obtain from working for wages. This can be used to advance

Table 5-1 Descriptive Statistics (mean values)

	Illiterate Farmers (1)	Literate Farmers (2)	Ratio of Means (2)/(1)
Income, Production and Profit:			
Total Income	504.5	775.1	1.54
Farm Income	290.5	449.9	1.55
Agriculture Production:	261.5	407.3	1.56
Cash Crops	(89.3)	(195.8)	(2.19)
Food Crops	(172.2)	(211.1)	(1.22)
Profit	223.7	312.0	1.39
Factors of Production			
Land Size (cuerda)	78.3	82.8	1.06
Land Value	69.1	93.3	1.35
Labor (man-day):	238.9	253.3	1.06
Family Labor	(199.8)	(171.3)	.86
Hired Labor	(39.1)	(82.0)	2.10
Cash Inputs	17.6	31.9	1.81
Indices of Efficiency and Factor Combinations:			
Production/Land Value	3.77	4.50	1.19
Profit/Land Value	2.89	3.14	1.09
Production/Labor	1.10	1.81	1.65
Labor/Land Value	4.14	3.60	.87
Cash Inputs/Land Value	.23	.33	1.45
Cash Inputs/Labor	.07	.11	1.57
Others:			
Wages Paid	.83	.83	1.00
Wages Earned	1.55	2.65	1.71
Family Work for Wages (man-days)	113.20	104.30	.92
% Family Labor to Total Farm Labor	84%	68%	.81
% Hired Labor to Total Farm Labor	16%	32%	2.00
Wage Income	182.9	244.0	1.33
% Wage Income to Total Income	36%	30%	.83
Income Per Capita	88.1	150.4	1.70
Number of Cases	323	187	

All values in quetzales.
Cuerda = .044 hectare.

the hypothesis that illiterate farmers, on the average having less access to land, are more concerned with providing household needs than with maximizing net monetary income. Here one is unable to use the above observations to conclude as to whether or not literate farmers are better managers than illiterate farmers, for objectives can be different: literate farmers trying to maximize profits and net farm income; illiterate farmers seeking to maximize food-crop production for household consumption.

However, on the average, literate farmers have larger landholdings and attain higher levels of farm production, which means that the possible differences in objectives between literate and illiterate farmers may be due, not to the fact that one group is more educated than the other, but to the fact that educated farmers also tend to be larger farmers. Large farmers may be able to be profit maximizers while small farmers are food production maximizers. Small farmers, concerned with providing for basic home food needs, may be loath to enter the labor market or to shift toward more profitable cash crops. Certain social and environmental circumstances can also explain the reluctance of small farmers to sell labor services into local labor markets, wage labor being traditionally more acceptable for landless household members.

Testing for the significance of literacy vis-à-vis managerial capability requires that we classify farmers according to goals which will then permit us to find out whether literacy does explain managerial differences within each group. The classification of farmers according to hypothetical goals is the subject of Part II (based on the analyses of Fisk, 1964, 1977; Nakajima, 1969; and A.K. Sen, 1966) and provides the rationale for grouping our Guatemalan farm-managers into three major groups.

Part II: Grouping Farmers according to Market Integration

Fisk and Nakajima describe development in rural subsistence economies as a process that develops over time, as people come to have progressive contact with the market; this, in turn, stimulates specialization and increases the value of cash income with respect to income-in-kind—mostly production of consumption food staples. The Fisk-Nakajima framework applies when there are no constraints on land and when cultural values are most important in explaining participation in labor and commodity markets. This is not true for our sample; we find land constraints are among the most significant determinants of scale of operations. These authors, however, offer rich material describing behavioral differences among farmers, which we will use here, considering that landholding size, rather than cultural differences, is the basis of differences in farmer behavior.

According to the Nakajima-Fisk (NF) model, subsistence economies develop through three phases. In the first "subsistence-unit" phase, farmers lacking contact with money markets produce staple goods for home consumption only. Allocation of working time and production depends only on the farmer's preferences as to income and leisure, and on constraints of fixed resources (labor only, in NF model). In the second phase, "subsistence with complementary cash income," farmers have some contact with the market and begin to value money income. Production begins to exceed immediate consumption needs, and production surplus is sold for specific cash income. Participation in the labor market often provides a way to earn additional money income, but home food production must be assured before labor will be allocated to any other income-earning activity. The last phase, "market integration with subsidiary food production," corresponds to a certain degree of market specialization. Farmers in this group allocate resources chiefly to marketed products, but may continue to produce food staples if this is seen as efficient. Participation in the labor market (buying and selling labor services) will vary according to farmers' criteria of efficiency rather than to any preference for production-income versus money-income. In this phase, farmers value monetary income per se and are indifferent with respect to its source.

In our study, land and associated risk-attitudes, together with social values, determine the transition between phases of the NF model. We classified farmers into three categories according to the degree of market integration: subsistence, semi-subsistence, and commercial. *Subsistence farmers* grow food for household consumption only and sell no crops. Income levels are low and constrained by size of landholdings; often these farmers sell labor services to complement their agricultural income. *Semi-subsistence farmers* grow food crops only, but they obtain a certain surplus which is sold in the market. *Commercial farmers* grow and sell both food and cash crops. The average landholdings of each group are: for subsistence farmers, between 39 and 48 units of quality land; for semi-subsistence farmers, between 66 and 86 units; and for commercial farmers, between 126 and 165 land units.

We can now undertake analysis of each of these three groups, in order to see whether, within each group, literate farmers still behave differently from illiterate ones, or whether disaggregation of the sample into these three groups wiped out most previously detected differences. Table 5-2 shows relevant production indices for each group.

The values given in Table 5-2 show that previous comments on the differences between literate and illiterate farmers in organizing production do not hold equally for each group, as now defined according to market integration and landholdings. Table 5-1, for example, indicated that literate farmers achieved higher levels of yield and profit per land-unit, used higher cash inputs per land, and lower labor-land combinations. Now, the advantage of literate farmers in obtaining higher production and profit per land is seen here for only two of the groups: semi-subsistence and commercial farmers. Regardless of literacy status, subsistence farmers attain approximately the same level of profit and yield, and use the same amount of cash inputs per land.

The second characteristic previously detected for literate farmers—substitution of cash inputs for labor—remains true for the three groups. Literacy continues, therefore, to be associated with use of cash-input-intensive combinations, whether due to management skills or to varying access to credit. This last factor is likely to be less important since landholding size is now partially controlled by having the farmers classified according to scale of operations.

Three additional remarks are worth making. First, literate farmers in subsistence groups obtain the same level of land productivity as illiterate farmers, using, however, 28 percent less labor per land unit but 80 percent more of cash inputs per man-day. If one assumes that both illiterate and literate farmers are equally efficient in maximizing profits, this means that either the relative price of cash inputs with respect to labor is 80 percent higher for illiterate farmers than for literate farmers, or that educated labor is 80 percent more efficient (see Technical Appendix for details).

The second observation concerns the use of land-labor combinations among literate and illiterate farmers in both the semi-subsistence and commercial groups. As the Technical Appendix shows in Note 3, this corresponds to profit-maximizing behavior, supporting the assumption that both groups operate under profit-maximization objectives. And last, any advantage literate farmers have in profit and yield per land (due to more intensive use of cash

Table 5-2 **Production Indices of Three Farmer Groups (mean values)**

	Subsistence			Semi-subsistence			Commercial		
	Illit. (1)	Liter. (2)	Ratio (2)/(1)	Illit. (3)	Liter. (4)	Ratio (4)/(3)	Illit. (5)	Liter. (6)	Ratio (6)/(5)
Production/Land	2.94	2.88	.98	4.27	5.64	1.32	5.66	7.33	1.30
Profit/Land	2.47	2.40	.97	3.83	4.76	1.24	4.51	5.33	1.18
Production/Labor	.73	1.10	1.50	1.34	2.36	1.76	1.48	1.79	1.21
Labor/Land	4.48	3.23	.72	3.95	3.68	.93	4.05	4.02	.99
Cash Inputs/Land	.18	.19	1.06	.19	.23	1.21	.46	.68	1.48
Cash Inputs/Labor	.04	.07	1.80	.08	.11	1.40	.13	.17	1.31
Land Value	42.80	45.60	1.07	66.90	88.20	1.30	142.70	149.30	1.05
% Hired Labor	8.00	8.00	1.00	11.30	26.20	2.38	25.80	41.80	1.62
Income Per Capita	63.70	108.30	1.70	89.80	136.00	1.52	147.30	224.30	1.52
No. Cases	140	56		129	83		54	48	

Land measured in standardized quality units.

inputs) is relatively higher among semi-subsistence than among commercial farmers. Within the latter group literate farmers use 48 percent more inputs (per land unit) to obtain 32 percent more yield (per land unit); for the former group, the corresponding values are 21 percent and 30 percent. The joint effect of literacy-cash inputs seems, therefore, to decrease with degree of commercialization.

In short, by disaggregating our sample according to market integration we came to the following conclusions:

(a) Literate farmers consistently use more cash-input-intensive combinations than illiterate farmers, regardless of market integration.

(b) Literate farmers tend to substitute cash inputs for labor, especially among subsistence farmers who attain the same land productivity as illiterate farmers with much less labor per land. This opens the possibility that, leaving aside differences in relative prices (of cash inputs with respect to price of labor), and holding everything else constant, educated farmers attain higher levels of labor productivity.

(c) Semi-subsistence and commercial farmers operate with the same labor-land ratio, supporting the hypothesis that their shared goal is profit maximization.

(d) Intensity of cash inputs increases with degree of commercialization; the joint effect of education and cash inputs seems, however, to decline with commercialization.

We conclude that disaggregation of farmers according to market integration is useful to our analysis, allowing finer identification of managerial differences between literate and illiterate farmers, differences which otherwise might be confounded with the influence of different objectives, or differences in size of landholdings. Our next task is to use econometric techniques to confirm or deny some preliminary hypotheses: Do literate farmers have an edge in reaching higher levels of production through the same factors of production? Are literate farmers more able to maximize profits, given their increased ability to adapt input combinations according to perceived market-factor prices? In technical terms, we refer to the first hypothesis as testing for *technical efficiency*, and the second as testing for *price or allocative efficiency*. These concepts are defined more precisely in Part III, which includes the functions to be estimated, and the econometric results.

Part III: Literacy and Farm Efficiency

As emphasized by Lau and Yotopoulos (1971, 1973), efficiency can be defined from various perspectives, two of which are noted here: technical and price (or allocative) efficiency. The first says that a farmer is *technically* efficient whenever (for a certain amount of production factors) he achieves the maximum possible amount of output. Thus farmer a will be more efficient (in technical terms) than farmer b if, for the same production factors, farmer a obtains higher ouput than does farmer b. On the other hand, one says that a farmer is *price* efficient if his input combinations are chosen so as to yield the maximum profit, that is, if the chosen level of each production factor is such that its marginal product equals its market price.

To illustrate these concepts, assume a fixed form of production function as

$$Y = F(L,T,I) \tag{5.1}$$

where Y is output, and L, I, and T, are labor, cash inputs, and land, respectively. Let us now consider a set of K production functions differing only by a scale factor, A_i, with $i = 1 \ldots, K$,

$$Y_i = A_i F(L, T, I) \tag{5.2}$$

One says that farmer i is *technically* more efficient than farmer j, if their production functions differ only by the scale parameter 'A', and A_i is greater than A_j. That is, with the same production factors, farmer i attains more output than farmer j by a factor A_i/A_j. Testing for the hypothesis that literate farmers are technically more efficient than illiterate farmers amounts, therefore, to testing for whether A_i/A_j is greater than 1, with i and j denoting literate and illiterate farmers, respectively.

For a production function such as in Equation (5.1), we say that price efficiency is achieved when the value of marginal product of each factor equals its market price. Thus, for a generic factor of production x,

$$\partial Y/\partial x = k_x p_x \tag{5.3}$$

If farmers do not achieve price efficiency, their choice of factor combinations fails to comply with (5.3), and the degree of price inefficiency can be expressed by

$$\partial Y/\partial x = k_x p_x \qquad (5.4)$$

where k stands for the inefficiency factor with respect to input x. Allowing for differences in price efficiency among farmers, one writes

$$\partial Y_i/\partial x_i = k_{xi} p_x$$

where k_{xi} is the inefficiency parameter of farmer i. Consequently, one can test whether farmers i and j differ in price efficiency by testing whether the parameters k_{xi} and k_{xj} differ among farmers. This test can be carried out either by deriving the factor marginal products from estimated production functions, or by estimating a normalized profit function (Yotopoulos and Lau, 1971; 1973), which allows for technical and price efficiency to be tested simultaneously.

Testing Technical Efficiency

The preliminary analysis that followed Tables 5-1 and 5-2 aimed to see whether literate farmers' higher levels of land productivity could be explained by the use of production factors in different combinations, thus leading us to conclude that literate farmers use greater cash inputs and less labor per unit of labor. To find out if this corresponds to greater *technical* efficiency of literate farmers (or less technical efficiency of illiterate farmers) demands that we ask whether illiterate farmers could obtain higher levels of land productivity with the *same* input combinations that they actually do use.

Since land was assumed fixed in the short run, our production function in Equation (5.2) can be expressed as

$$Y_i/T_i = A_i \, G(L_i/T_i, I_i/T_i) \quad i = 1 \text{ if farmer is illiterate} \qquad (5.5)$$
$$i = 2 \text{ if literate}$$

where $G(L/T, I/T) = F(L/T, 1, I/T)$, provided function $F(.)$ is homogeneous of degree one, that is, presents constant returns to scale. Our previous analysis, in fact, amounted to comparing the ratios Y/T, L/T, and I/T, among farmers with different literacy status. If these values were approximately the same, the scale parameter, A, also would be the same, and both groups would be seen as equal in terms of technical efficiency. This was not so; literate farmers used higher I/T's, lower L/T's, and obtained higher Y/T's than did illiterate farmers. We could not do much more than hint at possible explanations for this. In fact, to reach definite conclusions on technical differences between literate and illiterate farmers one has to assume something more specific about the form of the function $F(.)$.

Let us now assume that $F(.)$ is a Cobb-Douglas function, representing the technological possibilities of farmers, that can be written as

$$lnY = a + b_1lnL + b_2lnT + b_3lnI + b_4lnKA + b_5lnKB \qquad (5.6)$$
$$+ \Sigma c_i V_i + dR + \Sigma e_j Com_j$$

where Y, L, and T are agricultural production, labor, and land value, respectively; I represents cash inputs, KA and KB are animal capital and physical capital; V_i denotes the village that farmers come from with $i = 2,3,4$; R is a $(0,1)$ variable, equal to 0 if farmer is illiterate, and equal to 1 otherwise; and Com_j is another index variable taking on values of 0 or 1 denoting whether the farmer belongs to one of the commercialization groups.

Equation (5.6) was fitted to the overall sample and to five separate groups within the sample: literate, illiterate, subsistence, semi-subsistence, and commercial farmers. Coefficients estimated for v_i represent structural differences among villages; those estimated for r and e_j represent differences in the technological parameters described in the foregoing paragraphs. Table 5-3 shows regression coefficients obtained by Ordinary Least Square estimation. The following conclusions seem evident:

1. All the regression models seem to explain much of the variation in total farm production: between 68 percent and 74 percent, when a degree of commercialization enters the equation; and between 62 percent and 70 percent, when commercialization is left out. For most models, physical-input coefficients are significant at the 1 percent level of confidence, cash-input coefficients having the highest t-statistic values. Exceptions are labor in the semi-subsistence group (not significantly different from zero), and land and capital inputs among commercial farmers. Summation of coefficients varies between 0.95 and 1.1 showing, for the total sample and for literate and illiterate farmers, constant returns to scale; as for commercialization groups, the sum of factor coefficients goes from 0.85 in the subsistence group to 1.13 in the commercial group, denoting increasing

Table 5-3   OLS Estimated Coefficients of Production Functions by Group of Farmers

| Variables | Total Sample | | By Literacy Level | | | By Degree of Commercialization | | |
	(1)		Illiterate Farmers (2)	Literate Farmers (3)		Subsistence (4)	Semi-Subsistence (5)	Commercial (6)
LNLAB, Ln. Labor (man-days)	.291* (6.93)	.268* (6.09)	.256* (4.49)	.374* (4.29)	.310* (3.64)	.244* (3.49)	.064 (1.02)	.715* (5.67)
LNLD, Ln. Land Values	.284* (6.76)	.244* (4.21)	.304* (4.16)	.218* (2.15)	.157* (1.55)	.298* (3.10)	.375* (4.08)	.019* (.154)
LNINP, Ln. Cash Inputs	.285* (10.18)	.224* (7.47)	.205* (5.69)	.249* (4.88)	.249* (4.52)	.139* (2.34)	.205* (4.46)	.236* (3.63)
LNKA, Ln. Capital Animal		.039* (3.25)	.030* (2.14)	.072* (3.00)	.057* (2.59)	.044* (2.44)	.040* (2.35)	.007 (.269)
LNKB, Ln. Physical Capital	.207* (5.31)	.178* (4.45)	.131* (2.67)	.250* (3.52)	.234* (3.39)	.120 (1.71)	.279* (5.17)	.157 (1.74)
V2, Dummy = 1 If Village = 2		-.119 (-1.34)	-.202 (-1.94)	-.026 (.171)	-.035 (-2.09)	-.118 (-.849)	-.127 (-1.06)	-.203 (-.659)
V3, Dummy = 1 If Village = 3		.110 (1.06)	-.055 (-.434)	.372 (1.99)	.344 (1.91)	-.343 (-1.97)	.011 (.072)	.481 (1.43)
V4, Dummy = 1 If Village = 4		.103 (1.30)	.044 (.500)	.271 (1.53)	.211 (1.26)	.140 (1.228)	.056 (.509)	-.205 (-.505)
RWPA, Dummy = 1 If Literate Farmer	.176* (2.98)	.131* (2.34)				.127 (1.34)	.200* (2.53)	.016 (.135)
COM2, Dummy = 1 If Semi-subsistence Farmer		.499* (8.32)	.430* (6.32)		.620* (4.97)			
COM3, Dummy = 1 If Commercial Farmer		.626* (6.14)	.662* (5.39)		.577* (3.22)			
CONST, Constant	1.596* (5.91)	.160* (7.86)	1.80* (8.22)	1.52* (3.87)	1.76* (4.76)	1.92* (6.58)	2.76* (9.75)	.960 (1.54)
R^2	.683	.723	.736	.657	.702	.541	.616	.677
Adjusted R^2	.670	.717	.728	.642	.685	.519	.599	.646
ESS, Error Square Sum		167.3	89.4		74.4	60.56	58.9	28.3
D.F., Degrees of Freedom		498	312		174.0	186	202	92
Number of Cases		510	323		187	196	212	102

T-statistics in parentheses.
* Statistically significant at the 1 percent of confidence level.

returns with an increasing degree of commercialization or land-holding size, which is the most important determinant of degree of commercialization. The fitted function for the overall sample shows elasticities for land, labor, and cash inputs as approximately the same; estimates for illiterate farmers alone show that land has higher explanatory power; for literate farmers, on the other hand, labor explains most of the output variation. The fits for subsistence, semi-subsistence, and commercial farmers show some differences in the factor-elasticity estimates: Among subsistence farmers, factor elasticities are about at the same level; among semi-subsistence, land explains most of the output variation, while labor does this for commercial farmers.

2. Education coefficients are significant at the 1 percent confidence level in the whole sample regression, although this decreases somewhat when dummy variables, denoting degree of commercialization, enter the regression. According to the degree of market integration, the influence of education is at its peak among semi-subsistence farmers; it declines among subsistence farmers, and is insignificant for commercial farmers. Using a literate farmer's average years of schooling as 1.5 (as the sample indicates), the results show that, for the overall sample, one year of additional schooling is associated with 5.7 percent of increased agricultural output; among semi-subsistence farmers this value reaches 9 percent.

3. Testing for structural differences among literate and illiterate farmers (that is, for whether or not they have different production functions) leads to the impossibility of rejecting the hypothesis that literate and illiterate farmers have the same production function. Hence, literacy affects the technical scale parameter or equation (5.2), but not the physical input elasticities. That is, *illiterate and literate farmers have the same production function, but literate farmers are technically more efficient than illiterate farmers.*

4. Disaggregation of the total sample into three groups according to the degree of *commercialization* leads to important conclusions: Each group seems to have a different production function, and it is interesting to note that, while elasticity of cash inputs increases (both in magnitude and in its t-statistic) as one progresses from the subsistence to the commercial group, land elasticity is large among semi-subsistence and not significant among commercial farmers; however, labor elasticity, not significant in the semi-subsistence groups, is important for commercial farmers.

In short, the analysis of production functions indicates that literacy is related to higher levels of agriculture productivity and that education works as a scale parameter, shifting the production function without changing the output elasticities; that is, educated farmers seem to have relatively higher technical efficiency than their less-educated peers. Differences in commercialization (market integration) seem to be very important: Production functions were found structurally different between groups, education having the greatest influence on agricultural productivity of semi-subsistence farmers.

Simultaneous Testing for Technical and Price Efficiency

As discussed before, one way of testing for price efficiency is to compute the value of factor marginal products using the production-function estimates at mean values of actual factor combinations. For a Cobb-Douglas production function as estimated, this value—obtained by differentiation of $F(.)$ with respect to each factor input—is simply $b_x.Y/X$, where X is any factor of production and b_x is the corresponding coefficient estimate. If farmers do not differ in price efficiency, their marginal products should be the same, for the same factor prices. Table 5-4 shows the values of labor, land, and cash-input marginal products obtained for each group.

Table 5-4   Factor Marginal Productivity

| | Average Product | | | Marginal Product | | |
	Y/L	Y/T	Y/I	Labor	Land	Cash Inputs
Total Sample	1.36	4.40	15.2	.40	1.25	4.33
Illiterate	1.10	3.77	16.5	.32	1.07	4.70
Literate	1.81	4.50	14.1	.53	1.28	4.02
Subsistence	.84	2.92	18.7	.21	.09	2.60
Illiterate	.73	2.94	19.8	.18	.88	2.75
Literate	1.10	2.88	16.7	.27	.86	2.32
Semi-subsistence	1.74	4.80	22.5	.11	1.80	4.60
Illiterate	1.34	4.27	23.4	.09	1.60	4.80
Literate	2.36	5.64	21.6	.15	2.20	4.30
Commercial	1.62	6.44	11.9	1.16	.12	2.80
Illiterate	1.48	5.60	12.6	1.06	.11	2.97
Literate	1.79	7.33	11.2	1.28	.14	2.60

We see that: (1) Literate farmers operate at higher levels of labor and land marginal product (64 percent and 20 percent, respectively) than do illiterate farmers, pointing up the effect of using more cash inputs in increasing the marginal product of the other factors. (2) As for absolute price efficiency, that is, $dY/dX = P_x$, one observes that for an average daily wage of 0.83 quetzales, commercial farmers use less than the optimal amount of labor; and both subsistence and semi-subsistence farmers use labor in excess of what would be optimal for profit maximization; this may confirm our assumption that small farmers are less concerned with profit maximization than with providing for home food needs. (3) The fact that literate farmers operate at higher levels of labor-marginal product can also mean that the opportunity cost of family labor is 60 percent higher than the opportunity cost for illiterate farmers (see Table 5-1). (4) Nevertheless, among subsistence and semi-subsistence farmers educated farmers seem to be relatively more efficient though less efficient among commercial farmers. This analysis, however, is crude enough to keep us from drawing definite conclusions.

In fact, to depart from production-function estimates to analyze price efficiency is not the best method. Failure to maximize profits can be caused by failure to adapt factor combinations to their relative prices—so that the condition in Equation (5.3) holds—or by failure to obtain the maximum output from available production factors. That is, failure to maximize profits can be explained by price inefficiency, by technical inefficiency, or both.

To solve this problem, Yotopoulos and Lau proposed a method to test simultaneously for price and technical efficiency, based on the following (a more complete explanation is provided in Note 4, Technical Appendix):

1. A profit function derived from a Cobb-Douglas function that allows for differences in price efficiency, and can be written as

$$ln\ P = ln\ A^* + d\ D_2 + b_x^*\ ln\ p_x \qquad (5.7)$$

where P is normalized profit (profit normalized by output price); A^* is the scale parameter of our production function in Equation (5.2) now affected by the price inefficiency parameter, k_x of Equation (5.4); and b_x^* is derived from factor X elasticity affected by its price.

2. The Cobb-Douglas production function has the property that if farmers are equally efficient in price terms, their combination of factors will hold factor shares in total profit at the same level. If

farmers are equally, and also absolutely, efficient, this factor share is equal to b^*_x, the factor coefficient in the profit function of Equation (5.7).

Testing for differences in price efficiency (relative and absolute) among literate and illiterate farmers uses these two properties. First, one tests whether literate and illiterate farmers do keep the share of variable-factor cost at the same level; this means that, using labor as the variable factor of production, one must find out whether the share of labor costs (wL) in normalized profit (P) is constant across farmers, independent of their literacy. Next, one tests for whether this value (wL/P) equals the estimated labor coefficient, b^*, in the profit function of Equation (5.7). That is, one estimates two functions, the first being the profit function

$$ln\ P = ln\ A^* + dD_2 + b^*\ ln\ w \qquad (5.8)$$

and the second

$$wL/P = d_1\ D_1 + d_2\ D_2 \qquad (5.9)$$

where the D's are now dummy variables for literacy where D_1 equals one if the farmer is illiterate and zero otherwise; and D_2 equals one if the farmer is literate and zero otherwise.

Estimation of Equation (5.9) leads to testing if $d_1 = d_2$—that is, whether literate and illiterate farmers are equally efficient in price terms—and is carried out by performing a constrained estimation with $d_1 = d_2$; if the null hypothesis $(d_1 = d_2)$ cannot be rejected, then one proceeds by testing whether $d_1 = d_2 = b^*$ in (5.8). At this point one can observe the statistical significance of d in equation (5.8) which represents the technical efficiency of literate farmers compared with their illiterate counterparts.

We performed these tests for five different crops for which output prices exist, namely, corn, beans, tomato, chili, and *maicillo*. The estimation was carried out by the Zellner method, for which the results of unrestrained estimation, one restriction $(d_1 = d_2)$, and two restrictions $(d_1 = d_2 = b^*)$ are shown in Table 5-5.

Results were affected by the lack of variation in wage paid to hired labor. For all cases except beans, we could not reject the hypothesis that literate and illiterate farmers were equally efficient (or equally inefficient, in price terms). Moreover, the technical parameter A_i becomes insignificantly different from zero when profit functions are estimated under this method. A shortcoming of this analysis is that,

Table 5-5 Testing for Price Efficiency, Five Crops (T-statistics between parentheses)

Parameters	Beans			Corn		
	Unrest.	1 Restr.	2 Restr.	Unrest.	1 Restr.	2 Restr.
PROFIT FUNCTION						
ln A*	-2.89	-2.90	-3.13	.346	.380	.150
	(-1.86)	(-1.85)	(-3.81)	(.332)	(.364)	(1.54)
d (literacy)	.362	.209	.197	-.204	-.279	-.277
	(1.69)	(1.03)	(.979)	(.907)	(-1.29)	(-1.28)
a (ln w*)	-.766	-.801	-.877	-1.26*	-1.26*	-1.38*
	(-1.64)	(-.270)	(-4.64)	(-2.85)	(-2.84)	(-3.48)
b (ln LD)	.784*	.771*	.774*	.074	.074	.076
	(6.31)	(6.15)	(6.22)	(.548)	(.548)	(.555)
V_2 (viL2)	-.419	-.407	-.402	-.24	-.310	-.222
	(-1.34)	(-1.29)	(-1.29)	(-1.6)	(-1.97)	(-1.30)
V_3 (viL3)	-.183	-.208	-.176	-.458	-.357	-.500
	(-.310)	(-.350)	(-.304)	(-2.11)	(-.225)	(-.206)
V_4 (viL4)	-.366	-.370	-.356	-.577	-.579	-.584
	(-1.00)	(-1.09)	(-.989)	(-2.43)	(-2.35)	(-2.19)
LABOR DEMAND FUNCTION						
r_1 (D_1)	-1.33*	-.894*	-.877*	-1.26	-1.82	-1.38
	(-4.89)	(-4.32)	(-4.63)	(-2.16)	(-2.13)	(-3.48)
r_2 (D_2)	-.431	-.894	-.877	-.510	-1.82	-1.38
	(-1.54)	(-4.32)	(-4.63)	(-7.13)	(-2.13)	(-1.38)
F Computed		5.55	2.78	1.48		.907
Critical Values for 1% Level of Confidence		6.90	4.85	6.80		4.74
Critical Values for 5% Level of Confidence		3.95	3.10	3.90		3.05

Table 5-5 (continued)

Parameters	Tomato			Chili		
	Unrestr.	1 Restr.	2 Restr.	Unrestr.	1 Restr.	2 Restr.
PROFIT FUNCTION						
ln A*	2.99*	3.01*	3.09*	-.250	-.209	-.062
	(2.82)	(2.87)	(2.95)	(-.188)	(-.157)	(-.043)
d (literacy)	-.121	-.187	-.185	.179	.118	.031
	(-.37)	(-.58)	(-.58)	(.380)	(.250)	(.060)
a (ln w*)	-.058*	-.059*	-.504	-1.79*	-1.79*	-1.58*
	(-2.21)	(-2.23)	(-3.50)	(-3.32)	(-3.33)	(-2.79)
b (ln LD)	.676*	.677*	.691*	.575*	.574*	.605
	(3.55)	(3.54)	(3.73)	(2.22)	(2.22)	(2.12)
V_2 (viL2)	-1.24	-1.24	-1.27	.394	.392	.356
	(-1.42)	(-1.41)	(-1.44)	(.749)	(.745)	(.617)
V_3 (viL3)	—	—	—	—	—	—
	—	—	—	—	—	—
V_4 (viL4)	-1.25	-1.24	-1.29	.275	.271	.387
	(-1.13)	(-1.13)	(-1.17)	(.187)	(.185)	(.239)
LABOR DEMAND FUNCTION						
r_1 (D_1)	-.139	-.471	-.504	2.42	-.127	-1.58
	(-.626)	(-2.76)	(-3.50)	(.038)	(-.071)	(-2.79)
r_2 (D_2)	.884*	-.471	-.504	-2.29	-.127	-1.58
	(-3.55)	(-2.76)	(-3.50)	(.964)	(-.071)	(-2.79)
F Computed		4.96	2.55		1.81	1.32
Critical Values for 1% Level of Confidence		6.80	4.70		7.05	4.95
Critical Values for 5% Level of Confidence		3.89	3.05		3.90	3.14

Table 5-5 (continued)

Parameters	Maicillo		
	Unrestr.	1 Restr.	2 Restr.
PROFIT FUNCTION			
In A*	.989	1.09	−.359
	(.324)	(.355)	(−1.24)
d (literacy)	−.087	−.396	−.428
	(−.099)	(−.465)	(−.467)
a (ln w*)	.014	.004	−.653
	(.013)	(.004)	(−7.34)
b (ln LD)	.366	.352	−.211
	(1.07)	(1.02)	(.625)
V_2 (viL2)	−3.48*	−3.96*	−2.93
	(−2.16)	(−2.07)	(−1.73)
V_3 (viL3)	—	—	—
	—	—	—
V_4 (viL4)	−3.19	−3.52	−11.76
	(−.377)	(.414)	(−.198)
LABOR DEMAND FUNCTION			
r_1 (D_1)	−1.60	−.653	−.653
	(1.15)	(−.734)	(−.734)
r_2 (D_2)	−1.60	−.653	−.653
	(1.15)	(−.734)	(−.734)
F Computed		1.62	1.28
Critical Values for 1% Level of Confidence		7.62	7.50
Critical Values for 5% Level of Confidence		4.19	3.32

concentrated in individual crops, it does not allow for showing up the advantage of literate farmers who choose the best crop mix. This was, however, included in the production-function approach used to analyze technical efficiency, for variation in the dependent variable—value of farm production—included not only variation in production of each crop but also the effect of using different combinations of crops grown.

Conclusions

Table 5-6 summarizes the most important findings of this analysis. Two major conclusions can be briefly described as:

(1) Education is relevant in explaining differences in agricultural productivity. Literate farmers achieved higher levels of both land and labor productivity, partly due to more intensive use of chemical fertilizers, and partly because of a significant advantage in technical efficiency. This is particularly evident among semi-subsistence farmers, for whom a 9 percent increase in farm production is associated with an additional year of schooling.

(2) As for the influence of education on price efficiency, the analysis provided no definitive answers. This may be because our tests were based on the assumption of profit maximization and, as seen before, this is not true for many farmers; or because the data on wages did not provide enough variation to explain differences in allocative efficiency.

References

FISK, E. K. "The Response of Nonmonetary Production Units to Contact with the Production of a Market Surplus." *Economic Record 40* (1964).

FISK, E. K. "The Response of Nonmonetary Production Units to Contact with the Exchange Economy." *Agriculture in Development Theory*. New Haven: Yale University Press, 1977.

GRILICHES, Z. "Estimating Returns of School: Some Economic Problems." *Econometrica 45* (January 1977): 1–22.

JAMISON, D., and L. J. LAU. *Farmer Education and Farm Efficiency*. Baltimore: The Johns Hopkins University Press, forthcoming.

LAU, L., and P. YOTOPOULOS. "A Test for Relative Efficiency and Application to Indian Agriculture." *American Economic Review 61* (1971): 94–109.

LOCKEED, M.; D. JAMISON; and L. LAU. "Farmer Education and Farmer Efficiency—A Survey." In *Education and Income*, edited by Timothy King. Washington, D.C.: The Work Bank, 1980.

NAKAJIMA, C. "Subsistence and Commercial Family Farms—Some Theoretical Models of Subjective Equilibrium." In *Subsistence Agriculture and Economic Development*. Chicago: Aldine, 1969.

REYNOLDS, L. G. "Agriculture in Development Theory: An Overview." In *Agriculture in Development Theory* by E. K. Fisk. New Haven: Yale University Press, 1977.

SCHULTZ, T. "The Value of the Ability to Deal With Development." *Journal of Economic Literature 13* (1975): 872–876.

SEN, A. K. "Peasants and Dualism With and Without Surplus Labor." *Journal of Political Economy 74* (October 1966): 424–450.

YOTOPOULOS, P. and L. J. LAU. "A Test for Relative Economic Efficiency: Some Further Results." *American Economic Revue 63* (1973): 214–223.

Table 5-6   Education and Agriculture Productivity (Education Variable: Farmer's Literacy)

Farm Group	Dependent Variable	Coefficient Education's Influence on Farm Output	T-Statistics	R^2	Increase % in Production Related to One Year of Schooling*
All, N = 510	Agriculture production	.131	2.12	.689	5.69
	Farm production	.153	2.55	.689	6.72
	Value added	.309	3.77	.489	14.7
Subsistence Farms (N = 196)	Farm production	.127	1.34	.541	5.5
Semi-subsist. (N = 212)	Farm production	.200	2.53	.616	9.0
Commercial Farms (N = 102)	Farm production	.016	.0135	.677	0.6
Semi-subsist. and Commercial (N = 314)	Agriculture production	.156	1.93	.599	6.9
Corn Producers (N = 500)	Value of harvest Av. prices	.062	1.21	.617	2.6
Bean Producers (N = 273)	Value bean harv. Av. prices	.245	2.67	.623	11.3
Tomato Producers (N = 91)	Value of tomato production	.152	.80	.539	6.7
Chili Producers (N = 42)	Value chili production	.246	2.70	.669	11.3
Maicillo Producers (N = 114)	Value of maicillo produced	.150	1.00	.380	6.6
Sell Corn or Beans (N = 267)	Corn harvest	.095	1.46	.607	4.1
	Bean harvest	.327	3.27	.615	15.7
Sell Both Corn and Beans N = 44	Corn Harvest	.342	2.09	.618	16.6
	Bean Harvest	.252	1.24	.708	11.7

* Computed from $(e^b - 1)/D$

Appendix 5–1

DESCRIPTION OF THE VILLAGES

Available information allows us to describe the four rural villages for only one year, 1974. Some features thus cannot be generalized. For example, one cannot be sure that food staple sales are equally effective in most years, or whether 1974 was exceptionally good in terms of crop harvest, and thus enabled farmers to sell food crops. Other characteristics—such as land size, specialization cash crops, and performance of non-farming activities—can be seen as indices less dependent on the influences of weather, amount of precipitation, and so on. The description below focuses essentially on describing the people of the four study villages in terms of chief occupation, sources of income, kind of farming activities, and such variables as family size and education. It complements descriptions of the villages found in Chapter 2.

The body of data available from the RAND-Rockefeller files concerns 818 families in the four villages. Information about farming activities or other income sources is available for only 737 families; also, exclusion of families for whom values are missing for many farming variables reduced the total number of families to 716. Of these, 598 were agricultural, with access to land; members of the remaining families worked as wage laborers or carried out other activities such as small trade and craft work. Given our interest in analyzing the influence of education on farm production, the present description will focus on the 598 farm families.

Table A5-1.1 depicts some elements for the total sample and for each village considered here. Only 17.3 percent of the families depend entirely on farming income. Salaried work to complement farming income is carried out by 70 percent of the families. On the average, wages account for 40 percent of total income of farmers in

Table A5-1.1 Income Sources by Villages

Villages	All	#1	#2	#3	#4
Income Sources:					
Structure of Cases (%)					
Agriculture Only	17.3	14.7	27.7	5.4	17.3
Agric. and Salaries	48.2	65.9	56.4	13.8	48.2
Agric. and Activities	12.6	9.4	5.3	26.2	13.6
Agric., Sal., and Act.	21.9	10.0	10.6	54.6	20.9
TOTAL	100.0	100.0	100.0	100.0	100.0
Structure of Income (%)					
Agriculture Income:	45.5	32.3	53.6	53.9	36.7
(Consumed)	(24.4)	(24.8)	(21.6)	(26.8)	(26.6)
(Sold)	(21.1)	(7.4)	(31.7)	(27.1)	(10.1)
Non-Agriculture:	54.5	67.8	46.4	46.1	63.3
Wage Income	39.8	55.6	34.6	31.2	36.7
Others	14.7	12.2	11.8	14.9	26.6
Number of cases (farmers)	598	170	188	130	110
Total Cases in Villages	83.6%	85%	84.7%	74.3%	92.4%
Total Income	550.8	531.4	662.7	489.2	465.4
Income per Capita	131.9	136.7	167.5	111.4	88.7

these villages. The weight of non-farming income on total income varies among villages: For Villages 2 and 3, 54 percent of income comes from agricultural sources; in Villages 1 and 4, corresponding values are 32.3 and 36.7 percent, respectively. This is related to other indices concerning land productivity and farm produce. One sees (Table A5-1.2) that Villages 2 and 3 have higher levels of land productivity, use larger amounts of cash inputs per land unit, and the ratio of food staples to total produce is considerably lower than for Villages 1 and 4. The percentage of farm output sold also is consequently higher in Villages 2 and 3. The average size of land plots is quite small, 1.3 hectares. On the average, however, families hold more than one plot, which makes the average landholding equal to 2.8 hectares (79.9 cuerdas).

Agricultural production consists mainly of five crops: corn and beans (food crops), tomato and chili (cash crops), and *maicillo* (for animal feeding). Other products, as *ayoit* and yucca, are less important. Table A5-1.3 shows the structure of production and sales by

Table A5-1.2 Indices for Agriculture Production by Village

Village	Total	Vil. 1	Vil. 2	Vil. 3	Vil. 4
Average Extension of Land per Family (cuerdas)	68.6	97.23	83.17	36.8	70.3
Average Size of Parcel (cuerdas)	27.5	28.70	37.7	15.3	23.5
Average Number of Plots	2.5	2.90	2.1	2.3	2.8
Average Price of Land (quetzales/cuerdas)	2.0	1.13	2.7	3.7	.9
Average Productivity of Land (quetzales/cuerdas)	4.79	3.0	4.81	8.85	3.16
Corn and Beans in Total Agriculture Output	55%	84%	50%	33%	74%
Corn and Beans Sold (out of respective output)	16%	14.4%	20.4%	7.7%	14.2%
Agriculture Output Sold	45.2%	23.7%	53.6%	54.9%	27.2%
Agriculture Output Not Sold	54.8%	76.3%	46.4%	45.0%	62.8%
Labor-Land Ratio	2.9	3.08	3.24	2.5	2.65
Fertilizer-Land Ratio	.34	.16	.39	.55	.19
Hired Labor-Total Labor	21.1%	11.97%	19.9%	47.9%	10.1%
Productivity of Labor (Gross)	1.15	.95	1.14	1.64	.99
Productivity of Labor (Net)	1.04	.90	1.02	1.42	.92
Families Using Hired Labor	38.6%	34.1%	43.0%	47.8%	28.4%
Average Wage	.84	.75	.85	.87	.84

Table A5-1.3 Characterization of Four Guatemalan Villages: Production and Sales of Five Major Crops

Village	Families					Weight Total				
	All	1	2	3	4	All	1	2	3	4
Crops Grown:										
Corn	95.0%	89.4%	97.3%	84.0%	97.3%	42.2%	70.8%	33.9%	32.4%	48.6%
Beans	51.0	51.3	73.4	12.3	49.1	12.7	13.3	16.3	.5	25.3
Tomato	15.2	2.1	44.1	—	3.6	14.1	1.8	30.6	—	2.5
Chili	7.0	—	12.8	13.1	.9	20.0	—	16.7	48.5	1.8
Maicillo	19.1	30.7	2.1	.8	46.4	3.1	8.7	—	0.0	11.6
Others	21.7	13.2	14.4	41.5	21.8	7.9	5.4	2.2	18.5	10.1
Total	100.0%	100.0%	100.0%	100.0%	100.0%	100.0%	100.0%	100.0%	100.0%	100.0%
	(598)	(189)	(188)	(139)	(110)	(300.2)	(201.2)	(419.5)	(355.2)	(184.2)

Village	Farmers' Sales[b]					Sold/Produced[c] (%)				
	All	1	2	3	4	All	1	2	3	4
Crops sold:[a]										
Corn	32.0%	37.0%	42.6%	32.1%	7.0%	12.2%	14.6%	14.4%	8.1%	6.2%
Beans	25.5	9.5	34.8	12.5	35.1	28.5	11.5	33.3	6.3	31.1
Tomato	98.0	75.0	100.0	—	100.0	97.6	98.9	97.6	—	88.7
Chili	100.0	—	100.0	100.0	100.0	75.0	—	99.9	60.0	100.0
Maicillo	41.2	57.0	.7	—	27.0	32.9	61.8	6.7	—	18.9
Others	100.0	100.0	100.0	100.0	100.0	100.0	100.0	100.0	100.0	100.0
Total	71.4%	56.8%	73.0%	62.0%	100.0%	46.4%	20.6%	29.4%	50.3%	27.4%
	(363)	(96)	(136)	(79)	(52)	(110.7)	(81.4)	(343.3)	(293.9)	(107.2)

[a] Value of sales evaluated at the average selling prices.
[b] Farmers selling the crop as a percentage of farmers growing it.
[c] Percentage of sales to production of farmers selling the crop.

villages as observed in 1974. Most grow corn, 32 percent of farmers selling 12.2 percent of their production, on the average. As the major source of food in these villages, corn represents 42.2 percent of total agricultural production, reaching its highest level in Village 3 where corn is 70.8 percent of total farm production. Beans, chief source of protein in villages, holds second place. Roughly half the farmers grow some beans; among these, one fourth sell some bean production (on the average, 29 percent). Fewer farmers (15 and 7 percent, respectively) grow tomato and chili, essentially for sale. *Maicillo*, grown by 19 percent of the farmers, represents only 3 percent of total average produce. *Maicillo*, however, is sold by 40 percent of those who cultivated it and who, on the average, sold 33 percent of their *maicillo* crops. Of all farmers, 20 percent plant other crops for sale; these crops represent around 8 percent of total produce.

Sales and salaried work yield a substantial amount of cash income, which makes these populations very different from subsistence-level farmers of the Nakajima-Fisk model. Adding sales, salary income, and income from other activities (such as small trade, arts and crafts) makes cash income represent, on the average, 75 percent of total income for this sample.

Hiring labor seems to be a common practice in most villages: 38.7 percent of farmers hire some labor, Villages 2 and 3 being those where hired labor is more heavily used (43 and 48 percent of farmers, respectively). In Village 3 total hired labor represents 48 percent of total labor input; in the remaining villages the average is less than 20 percent. This is consistent with the fact that Village 3 has the largest proportion of landless, non-farming families (25.7 percent).

Finally, education and family variables are shown in A5-1.4. Both family size and age of average farmer are quite similar across villages. Amount of schooling differs considerably among villages, however, though the average of educational grades is very low for all. Village 2 has low rates of literacy and grade attainment, although male household heads here report more literacy. On the average, males completed fewer grades than females. Figures on educational grades and literacy indicate no consistent relation between literacy and grades; for example, in Villages 1 and 2, male household heads have less schooling, but are likely to read and write better than females; conversely, Village 1 has the highest rate of male literacy, but in Village 3 males show the largest amount of schooling (al-

Table A5-1.4   Education and Family Variables by Village

Village	All	#1	#2	#3	#4
Family:	4.65	4.57	4.69	4.36	5.12
N. of People Present	4.60	4.48	4.58	4.29	5.00
N. of Minors	1.38	1.53	1.35	1.20	1.43
Age Mother	35.5	37.9	32.8	36.7	34.6
Age Father	34.2	34.1	35.8	31.2	35.5
Read and Write:[a]					
Mother	.39	.57	.25	.35	.39
Father	.32	.98	.39	.29	.33
Av. Family[b]	.80	.88	.70	.91	.68
Education (grades):					
Mother	.72	.90	.55	.75	.65
Father	.54	.43	.55	.76	.39
Av. Family[b]	1.27	1.35	1.04	1.68	1.06

[a] Average of points according to: 0 = cannot read and/or write; 1 = can read and/or write a little; 2 = can read and write well.
[b] Average computed for the members of the family age 7 or more.

though less than one year). Ability to read and write was tabulated by asking whether a person could read and write, rather than by testing. Indices were computed as an average of three values—0 if unable to read and write, 1 if reads and writes a little, and 2 if reads and writes well. When we regrouped into just two categories, using 0 for the two first categories and 1 for people who read and write well (Table A5-1.5), the results are more striking as far as village differences are concerned.

Table A5-1.5   Male Literacy Using 0, 1 Scale

Villages	All	#1	#2	#3	#4
Literacy of Males	.366	.362	.164	.525	.258

This confirms the relatively higher level of literacy in Village 3 and the lowest position of Village 2. Recalling that Villages 2 and 3 showed the highest land and labor productivity, one must conclude that these simple indices cannot prove anything about the size and direction of the influence of education on agricultural production. More complete analysis must be carried out in order to disentangle the effects of education from other factors that affect the productivity levels of these Guatemalan farmers.

A Word on Poverty in the Villages

Predominantly poor on the average (income per capita in 1974 was around $132), these villages also show a substantial degree of internal inequality. In terms of land distribution, the upper quintile of farmers controls more than 40 percent of the land. As for total income, wages and other income sources compensated for a small part of the skewed distribution in land; even so, 5 percent of the wealthiest families received 25 percent of the income. Gini coefficients computed for these two variable distributions were 0.555 and 0.495 respectively. Total agriculture production was equally highly concentrated—more than 32 percent accruing to the top quintile of the distribution.

The direct consequence of such inequality of both means of production and of income is that a considerable number of families lie below the poverty level (as defined by local standards). The average wage for all four villages lies at the lower limit of acceptable annual income for a family of 4.8 persons (approximately 220 quetzales). A second poverty measure was computed by estimating the cost of buying basic food products (corn and beans) at average village prices. This amounts to 45.1 quetzales per person per year for 220 kg corn and 39 kg beans per person per year. For an average 4.8-person family, the computed poverty level equals 207.5 quetzales per year in 1974 prices.

Disregarding other living expenses and using these income levels to define a poverty level, we can conclude that 35 percent lie below the poverty level. Consequences in terms of child malnutrition and in poor school attendance and performance are predictable. Table A5-1.6 depicts some indicators for the two groups of families divided according to their relative position with respect to the poverty level, here measured in terms of income per capita (45 quetzales/year) to control for the effect of family size.

Table A5-1.6 presents the profile of poverty: low levels of education (or at least relatively lower), small landholdings and more family farms, as opposed to commercial farms, either cultivating land owned by the family or by sharecropping. Meanwhile, poor families have fewer children than "all the others" (1.25 and 2.15, respectively), which may result from poverty itself or from the slightly higher average age of household head.

Table A5-1.6   The Profile of Poverty in the Four Rural Communities, 1974 (Percentage)

	Poor Families	All Others
Age of Head of Household:		
14–29	15	19
30–60	70	64
61+	15	17
Education of Head of Household:		
Literate	26	43
Illiterate	74	57
Educational Grades Household Head:		
0	72	54
1–2	12	19
3–4	11	21
5+	5	8
Position in Occupation of Head of Household:		
Employer (hiring wage labor)	3	20
Self Employed	31	25
Share Cropper	51	34
Wage-laborer in Community	9	11
Employed Outside Community	6	10
Total Land Exploited:	(44.4)	(77.8)
Nuclear Land	61	71
Extended Family Land	9	7
Rented Land	21	19
Municipal Land	9	3
Sources of Income:	(211)	(713)
Agriculture Income	48	45
Wages	36	40
Activities, Arts and Crafts	16	15
Number of Children 0–10:		
0	30	19
1–2	34	29
3–4	27	38
5+	8	15
Number of cases	164	430

Appendix 5–2

TECHNICAL NOTES

Note 1: Maximization of Income, Profits, and Production

Let us assume that farm household income, E, is the sum of farm income E_f and wages income, E_w

$$E = E_f + E_w \qquad (A5.1)$$

Farm income, E_f, in turn is evaluated as the value of farm production Y, and wages income is equal to the amount of household labor working for wages, L_w^h, times average wage of household labor w^h.

$$E_w = L_w^h \cdot w^h \qquad (A5.2)$$

Farm production is a function of available factors of production, land, T, labor, L, and cash inputs, I, and can be written as

$$Y = F(L, T, I) \qquad (A5.3)$$

where F is a "well-behaved" function, such that each factor has positive but decreasing marginal productivities, and factor marginal product increases with the amount of any other factor. That is,

$$f_L, f_T, f_I > 0$$

$$f_{LL}, f_{TT}, f_{II} < 0$$

and $\qquad\qquad\qquad\qquad\qquad\qquad\qquad\qquad (A5.4)$

$$f_{LT}, f_{LI}, f_{TI} > 0$$

Farm labor is the sum of family labor allocated to farm working, L_f^h, plus hired labor L^o,

$$L = L_f^h + L^o \tag{A5.5}$$

hired labor being paid an average wage, w^o. Using these expressions, one writes the maximization problem of net household income as

$$\text{Max:} \quad p_y F(L,T,I) - w^o L^o + w^h \cdot L_f^h$$
$$\text{subj:} \quad \text{(i)} \ T = \overline{T}$$
$$\text{(ii)} \ L = L_f^h + L^o$$
$$\text{(iii)} \ L^h = L_f^h + L_w^h \tag{A5.6}$$

The problem is solved by maximizing a function as

$$Z = p_y F(L,T,I) - w^o L^o + w^h \cdot L_f^h - \lambda_1(T - \overline{T})$$
$$- \lambda_2(L - L_f^h - L^o) - \lambda_3(L^h - L_f^h - L_w^h) \tag{A5.7}$$

which holds as first conditions for a maximum

$$f_{L^o} = w_o/p_y$$
$$f_{L_f^h} = w^h/p_y \tag{A5.8}$$
$$f_I = p_I/p_y$$

That is, maximization of net income implies the use of family labor in farming until its marginal product equates family market wage, w^h; and hired labor up to the point where labor marginal product equates the wage rate paid to hired labor, w^o. If family wage were the same as hired-labor wage, the farmer would first use family labor and then hired labor, up to the point at which $f_L = w^o = w^h$; if family wage, w^h, is higher than hired labor wage, w^o, hired labor can substitute for family labor, which is then allocated to the labor market: $L_w^h = L_f - L_f^h(w^h)$, where $L_f^h(w^h)$ is the amount of L_f^h at which $f_{L^h} = w^h$.

Note 2

If total net household income is the sum of net farm income and wage income,

$$E = E_f + E_w$$

maximization of E implies maximization of E_f, net farm income, and of E_w, wage income.

Note 3

For example, for a production function such as $y = f(l,t,i)$, if $f(.)$ is homogenous of the first degree, then $y = t.g(l/t, i/t)$, and marginal product of labor, $\partial y/\partial l$, is given by $\partial g/\partial (l/t)$, holding i/t constant. Assuming land constant in the short run, optimality conditions for both farm groups imply that firms will operate at the same level of labor-marginal product; this, ultimately, will be the wage rate practiced in the village. As for labor-land ratio (l/t), the optimal labor-land ratio, $(l/t)^*$, will be such that

$$g'(l/t_i)^* = g'(l/t_j)^*$$

for all i and j farms, since $g'(\ )$ is the same for all farms, the optimal $(l/t)^*$ will also be the same. With land fixed in the short run, $t_i = \bar{t}_i$, optimal labor inputs will be determined as

$$l_i^* = \bar{t}_i(l/t)^*$$

The amount of hired/sold labor services then would depend on the amount of labor available in the family, l_i^f, and the optimal amount l_i^*. Farmers will hire labor if l_f is less than l^*, and otherwise will sell.

Since groups differ in wage perceived in the labor markets—such as literate farmer members obtaining, on the average, wages 60 percent higher than the illiterate—the amount of family labor available for farming activities will be determined in the function of this wage w_i^*, $L_i^*(w)$: $\partial y/\partial l_i^* = w_i^*$. Optimal labor-land ratio will be a function of the minimum wage $\bar{w}$,

$$(l/t)^*: \partial g(l/t)^* = \bar{w}$$

and labor inputs by $l* = (l/t)* \; \bar{t}$. Labor will be hired or sold whenever family labor is less or greater than the optimal $l*$:

$$l_h(s) = l* - l_f^*(w*) = t.(l/t)* - l_f^*(w*)$$

Note 4: Testing Technical and Price Efficiency

For a complete description of the method summarized below, see Yotopoulos and Lau (1971).

Let us recall some of the definitions mentioned in Part III. Price efficiency exists when the farmer matches the marginal product of a given input with its price. For a function $y = f(x)$, price efficiency will be obtained whenever $f_x = p_x/p_y$. Conversely, one can define an index of price inefficiency as k^i, and write $f_x = k^i(p_x/p_y)$ as the maximization profit rule of a farmer i who perceives the current prices affected by an error k^i. If any two farmers have the same error k, then their relative price efficiency will be equal although both might be inefficient in operating their farms. If $k^i = k^j = 1$, both farmers will be absolutely efficient in terms of price or allocative efficiency. Since farmers can differ in technical constants a_i, as seen before, a simultaneous test for $a_i = a_j$ and $k_i = k_j = 1$ has to be carried out.

For a Cobb-Douglas production function as

$$Y = AL^{b_1}T^{b_2} \tag{A5.9}$$

Lau and Yotopoulos show that using duality theory leads to a variable profit function as follows:

$$P = P(w,T) = A^{(1-b_1)^{-1}} (1 - b_1)^{-\alpha}w^\alpha T^\beta \tag{A5.10}$$

where P is the normalized variable profit, w is the normalized wage rate,

$$\alpha = -b_1(1 - b_1)^{-1} \quad \text{and} \quad \beta = b_2(1 - b_1)^{-1}.$$

Variable profit is a decreasing function of the wage rate, w, and an increasing function of fixed factors—land. If farmers vary in technical efficiency, that is, $A_i \neq A_j$, one can substitute A_i for A in Equation A5.10; if, besides that, they also vary in price efficiency, $k_j \neq k_i$, the correspondent profit function is, as derived by those authors,

$$P_i = A_i^* w^\alpha T^\beta \tag{A5.11}$$

$$A_i^* = A_i^{(1-b_1)-1} (1 - b_1/k_i)(k_i)^{-\alpha} b_1^{-\alpha} \tag{A5.12}$$

The goal is to test whether or not $A_1 = A_2$ (where 1 denotes illiterates and 2 denotes literate farmers) by using a dummy variable to estimate A_2^*/A_1^*. The test will not work if $k_2 \neq k_1$ because the ratio A_2^*/A_1^* involves the constants k_1 and k_2, as follows:

$$\frac{A_2^*}{A_1^*} = \left(\frac{A_2}{A_1}\right)^{(1-b_1)-1} \left(\frac{1 - b_1/k_2}{1 - b_1/k_1}\right)\left(\frac{k_2}{k_1}\right)^\alpha \tag{A5.13}$$

If $k_2 = k_1$, however, the ratio simplifies to the following:

$$A_2^*/A_1^* = (A_2/A_1)(1 - b_1)^{-1} \tag{A5.14}$$

Hence, we must test $k_2 = k_1$ first. To do so, Yotopoulos and Lau exploit a convenient property of the Cobb-Douglas function. When factor prices vary, quantities adjust to keep factor shares constant. The same is true for the ratio of variable factor costs to variable profit. Suppose a farm responds efficiently to the wage rate, that is, $k_i = 1$. Then

$$-wL/P = -b_1(1 - b_1)^{-1} = \alpha. \tag{A5.15}$$

But, if farmers act as if wage rate is $k_i w$, then their ratio $k_1 wL/P$ will be constant as w varies, not wL/P. We do not observe $k_1 w$, but the authors show that when $k_i \neq 1$,

$$-wL/P = (1 - b_1)(k_i(1 - b_1/k_i))^{-1} = \alpha_i. \tag{A5.16}$$

This equation defines α_i. One can, therefore, test for $k^i = k^j$ by finding out if the ratio of the observed wage bill to variable profit is significantly different for illiterate and literate farmers. This can be done by means of

$$-wL/P - a^1 D^1 = a^2 D^2$$

where D^1 and D^2 are $(0,1)$ variables denoting illiterate $(D^1 = 1)$ and literate farmers $(D^2 = 1)$.

If the test shows equal relative price efficiency across groups, we can proceed to test absolute price efficiency and relative technical efficiency with the Cobb-Douglas profit function.

The two profit functions are

$$P_2 = A_2^* \, w^\alpha T^\beta \qquad\qquad (A5.17)$$

$$P_1 = A_1^* \, w^\alpha T^\beta \qquad\qquad (A5.18)$$

If one replaces A_1^* in (A5.18) by $A_1^*(A_2^*/A_1^*)$, one can estimate (A5.18) by means of

$$ln \, P = ln \, A^* + d \, D_2 + \alpha ln \, w + \beta \, ln \, T \qquad\qquad (A5.19)$$

where $d = ln \, (A_2^*/A_1^*) = (1/1 - b_1) \, ln \, (A_2/A_1)$. If d is significantly different from zero, then A_2 and A_1 are not equal. We can also test absolute price efficiency because if $k_2 = k_1 = 1$, then $\alpha_1 = \alpha_2 = \alpha$, as can be seen by inspecting the equation defining α in (A5.15).

Chapter 6

EDUCATION, FAMILY ECONOMIC PRODUCTION, AND FERTILITY: THE CASE OF RURAL AND SEMI-URBAN GUATEMALA

by Mari S. Simonen

This chapter summarizes analyses of socioeconomic and attitudinal determinants of fertility in rural and semi-urban Guatemala.* Fertility is defined as the number of children-ever-born irrespective of how many survive. Fertility is distinguished from fecundity in that fecundity refers only to the physiological capacity to conceive and bear children. We focus on how literacy in female heads of household, and familial economic production (wealth, mode of production, and income), affect the number of children-ever-born to the female head of household.

We ask whether literacy in the female, along with familial economic production, affects fertility and, if so, how and why, in the context of the communities under study. In addition, we want to try to discover what other factors may explain individual fertility in these communities.

Underlying this work is the need to understand why people in

---

* Note that data used here are from the four *rural* communities of the INCAP data base *and* from two *semi-urban* communities (from the RAND data base, to be described in this chapter). The present chapter presents in a summarized manner results developed in greater detail in Simonen, 1980.

less-developed countries (LDCs) are having a given number of children, so that women will be better able to choose when to bear and rear children, and also so that we can contribute to the design of more responsible population policies. Although the education-fertility relationship has received much attention in demographic research, it remains unclear whether and why individual education (particularly in the very first few years) affects fertility in countries with low levels of overall literacy (Cochrane, 1978). The effect on fertility of familial economic production has been looked at mainly as an income-fertility relationship—that is, as income of family increases, does fertility decrease or increase?—less work has been done on the potentially important effects on fertility of wealth and mode of production (McGreevey and Birdsall, 1974; Simon, 1974 and 1976; MacFarlane, 1978). Wealth here refers to ownership of means of production (land, machinery, tools, animals, dwellings, etc.), consumer durables (house, vehicles, radio, etc.), and other assets (stocks, bonds, real estate, savings, etc.). Mode of production refers mostly to the manner and degree in which a family/household is integrated into wider economic markets as suppliers of products or labor, or as buyers of wage labor (Deere and deJanvry, 1978).

Whether we are interested in designing more effective population policy (in order to produce a rapid decline in population growth), or in making reproduction truly a matter of choice, more knowledge is needed about how socioeconomic factors (such as literacy and familial production) affect fertility.

Since fertility is defined as the number of children-ever-born, our emphasis will be on the "stock" aspect of fertility—that is, the number of children born to a female at a given time in her life (Namboodiri, 1972 and 1974; Cochrane, 1978). The "stock" model of fertility is to be contrasted with the "flow" model, in which one considers fertility from the point of view of adding/not adding another child to a given "stock."

The data come from a series of cross-sectional household surveys administered in 1975–1976 in the same four rural Guatemalan communities in which INCAP carried out the nutrition experiment as well as in two semi-urban communities near Guatemala City. All six communities are part of the Ladino, rather than the Indian, culture. (See Chapter 2 for a fuller description of the four rural villages and a later section of the present chapter for a description of the two semi-urban villages.)

Theoretical Framework and Methodology

The analytical work in this chapter centers on estimating a structural equation model of fertility determinants. The model (which will be shown later in Figures 6-1 and 6-2) represents postulated causal relationships among variables.

The model is based on extensive conceptual work in different theories of fertility determinants. Only a brief summary of the model can be presented here. (For a more complete review of the theoretical framework, see Simonen, 1980.) It is hypothesized that individual literacy and familial economic production (income, wealth, and mode of production), together with female labor-force participation, affect family type (extended or nuclear), child mortality, and community characteristics—for instance, availability of family planning services affects fertility through three intervening variables: (a) family planning knowledge, attitudes, and practice (KAP); (b) male/female communication; and (c) child utility.

Theories and findings from psychology and sociology emphasize that education and other socioeconomic variables (such as income, wealth, and mode of production) not only improve access to family-planning information and services, but also allow people to make more informed decisions about family planning. Additionally, education is thought to contribute to more positive attitudes toward the idea of spacing births and limiting family size (Berelson, 1966; Cochrane, 1978). Some theoretical and empirical evidence supports the hypothesis that the combined effect of family planning knowledge, attitudes, and practice (KAP) has a fertility-reducing effect (Celade, 1972; Sear, 1975; Williams, 1976; Cochrane, 1978), but the underlying theoretical argument is not well developed. The argument is simply that favorable attitudes toward, knowledge about, and use of contraception help parents control fertility (Williams, 1976). Moreover, evidence is accumulating to suggest that family-planning KAP may be a significant influence on fertility only after the motivation to have no more children has been reached—that is, generally after the family has the number of children (or at least the number of boys) judged necessary to assure a given number of surviving children when parents have reached retirement age (Wyan and Gordon, 1971; McGreevey and Birdsall, 1974; Cochrane, 1978).

Social psychological theories of interpersonal decision-making emphasize the importance of social-exchange processes within the family in determining family size and fertility (Hill, *et al.*, 1955; Bagozzi and Van Loo, 1978). These theories assume further that education and other socioeconomic variables operate mainly through the mechanism of social exchange within the family, although neither theory nor empirical evidence provides more information. There is evidence, however, that both education and socioeconomic variables are positively correlated with levels of social exchange within the family (Cochrane, 1978, Chapter 5).

Theories of Fertility

Economic, sociological, anthropological, and psychological theories of fertility all deal with the role played by the real and perceived values of children in determining fertility (Davis, 1955; Leibenstein, 1957; Nag in Fawcett, 1972; Hoffman and Hoffman, 1973; Cassen, 1976). Psychologists tend to focus on the psychoiogical value of children to parents; economists stress the economic/utilitarian value (contribution to income, and as old-age security); and sociologists emphasize the perceived long-term societal value of children. These theories further hypothesize that societal-level variables as well as individual education, income, wealth, and production-pattern affect child utility; that is, as socioeconomic conditions improve, the values (utilities) of children are affected, in that economic benefits provided by offspring tend to decrease while both direct and indirect costs tend to increase. Theoretical work on the effects of mode of production on fertility stresses that the number of children in a family is largely a reflection of parents' need for children to help in family economic activities. The need for children's help in turn is influenced by how the family produces its livelihood (MacFarlane, 1978; Deere and deJanvry, 1978).

Our fertility model hypothesizes that the socioeconomic variables affect family planning KAP and male/female communication similarly in the rural and in the semi-urban area. The effects of literacy, land-ownership, income, and female labor-force participation on perceived child utility and on fertility, however, are hypothesized to vary by rural versus semi-urban area.

We hypothesize that the net direct and indirect effects on fertility of the socioeconomic variables mentioned above are positive in the rural sample and that they are negative in the semi-urban sample.

(In the path model, direct effects are those that affect fertility directly without first affecting one of the model's intervening variables—family planning KAP, male/female communication, and perceived child utility. Indirect effects on fertility are those operating through the intervening variables. Positive effect refers to increasing fertility; negative effect means reducing fertility.) Different effects are expected between rural and semi-urban areas. In the rural context, improved socioeconomic status may increase parents' capacity to afford children but may not decrease the need for children's help. In the semi-urban context, the changing socioeconomic context and production pattern of families tend to decrease children's utilities (benefits) while increasing their costs to parents (Goldstein, 1972; Bindary *et al.*, 1973; McGreevey and Birdsall, 1974; Simon, 1974; Davidson, 1977).

The effect on fertility of family type (nuclear versus extended) is hypothesized to operate both through perceived child utility and male/female communication. A move toward a nuclear family is hypothesized to decrease the net value of children due to an increase in their costs and decrease in value (Leibenstein, 1957; Schultz, 1969; Simon, 1974). Similarly, a move toward extended family is hypothesized to increase the net value of children. How family type affects male/female communication is left unspecified because of limited theoretical and empirical evidence.

And last, we hypothesize that child mortality has a positive direct effect on fertility; this follows the theoretical work of economists and others on child-survival hypothesis and replacement behavior (Schultz, 1976; Preston, 1978). Although a controversy exists about how much child mortality does affect fertility, ample evidence supports a positive relationship (CICRED, 1974; McGreevey and Birdsall, 1974). The reason for modeling child mortality as an exogenous rather than as an intervening variable is mainly practical; limits had to be set on the focus and number of relationships examined in this study.

Methodology*

The main analytic technique used in this study is structural equation model estimation by means of ordinary least squares (OLS) regres-

---

* See also Technical Appendix at end of chapter.

sion method, path analysis (Duncan, 1975). Since OLS regression is used, the basic OLS assumptions are made. In addition, for OLS to yield unbiased and efficient estimates of structural parameters, and for these parameters to be identified, it is assumed that error terms in a recursive system of equations (such as our fertility model) are uncorrelated.

The model is estimated for female respondents aged 14+ living in union with a male at the time of the interview. The model is estimated separately by rural and semi-urban subsamples.

In structural equation analysis the causal effect of a one-unit change in a predictor variable on a dependent variable is represented as a parameter. In order to obtain unbiased estimates of the structural equation parameters, the model has to be correctly specified—that is, the causal ordering of the variables and choice of variables themselves should reflect reality accurately.

Since the model is assumed to be recursive, the parameters can be uniquely determined from observed data. A recursive model is a hierarchical model in which the errors in different equations are assumed to be uncorrelated with each other. A hierarchical model is one in which all causal linkages run "one way."

The major advantage of structural equation models is that they allow the effect of a predictor variable (for example, literacy) on a dependent variable (for example, fertility) to be separated into a direct effect, and one or more indirect effects which are transmitted through intervening variables (for example, family-planning KAP).

Since cross-sectional data are used, one should be cautious about interpreting the observed effects. This is especially relevant for attitudinal variables in the study, which were collected contemporaneously with fertility information. In addition, we offer a word of caution about possible reciprocal causation between certain variables in our model, for example, child mortality with fertility and female labor force participation with fertility. In addition, correlation and/or multicollinearity among error terms in equations cannot be entirely ruled out.

Characteristics of the Sample

The *sample* consists of a total of 847 female respondents (578 rural and 269 semi-urban) aged 14+ at the time of interviews in 1975–1976. These 847 respondents were living in union then (consensual or legal) with a male, or had been in union before. Note, however, that the *models* presented in this report are estimated only for females actually living in union with a male at the time of the interviews. The unit of analysis is the individual *female* head of household as she interacts variously with the male head of household, the rest of the family and household, and others in the community of residence.

In addition to the four rural villages, described in Chapter 2, the present analysis of fertility uses data from two semi-urban communities, which will be described as Villages 5 and 6. These two semi-urban communities are located about twenty minutes (driving time; city buses run regularly) from Guatemala City in a fairly industrial and rapidly urbanizing zone. The combined population is about 4,800 people (Butz *et al.*, 1975). The semi-urban communities represent a transitional zone from the country to the city. They share many socioeconomic and cultural characteristics of the capital, and many inhabitants work in Guatemala City. Houses are of better quality and of more formal construction than in the rural communities. Fewer houses have dirt floors; over half the houses have electricity; and practically all have some sanitary facilities. Streets are paved and cars, buses, motorcycles, and bicycles are a common sight.

Table 6-1 presents selected measures that describe the four rural villages and the two semi-urban communities. We see that the mean per capita income was around 200 quetzales in the semi-urban communities in 1974, that is, twice that in the rural communities. Major source of income is wage work: About three fourths of total 1974 household income in the semi-urban area was from wages. A larger percentage of females in the semi-urban area work as domestics, merchants, and factory workers than do women in the rural area. Inhabitants in the semi-urban communities have more schooling on average than their rural counterparts. Both parity and child mortality are somewhat lower in the semi-urban communities. In the semi-urban area overall, socioeconomic differences between families are apparent, for the upper quintile of families received 32 percent of the income.

The two semi-urban communities differ from each other in that one is more agriculturally based (Village 6) than the other. They also differ in the fact that Village 5 includes a larger proportion of young recent migrants from the rural areas; people here tend to have more contact with Guatemala City than do those in Village 6 (Clark, 1979). Male wages in Village 5 are higher than in Village 6.

Table 6-1 Mean and Standard Deviation of Selected Demographic and Socioeconomic Variables Describing Sample

	Rural Village (Number)					Semi-urban Community (Number)		
	1	*2*	*3*	*4*	*All*	*5*	*6*	*All*
Female Age:								
$\bar{x}$	39	35	38	36	37	34	35	34
SD	15	12	15	14	14	10	14	13
N	172	167	137	102	578	114	155	269
Male Age:								
$\bar{x}$	42	39	42	41	41	38	40	39
SD	12	11	15	13	13	9	14	12
N	134	140	101	89	464	107	128	235
Family Size:								
$\bar{x}$	5.11	5.25	4.84	5.54	5.17	5.60	4.90	5.20
SD	2.28	2.28	2.28	2.30	2.28	2.10	2.02	2.08
N	161	159	128	100	548	113	155	268
Children Ever-Born:								
$\bar{x}$	5.70	5.92	5.01	6.39	5.72	4.74	4.57	4.64
SD	3.38	3.91	3.14	3.91	3.61	2.58	2.97	2.81
N	172	167	137	102	578	114	155	269
Completed Parity (age 45–55):								
$\bar{x}$	8.13	8.86	8.11	9.71	8.62	6.50	7.29	7.00
SD	3.37	3.55	3.85	4.16	3.67	2.37	2.14	2.22
N	30	22	18	17	87	10	17	27

Table 6-1 (Continued)

	Rural Village (Number)					Semi-urban Community (Number)		
	1	2	3	4	All	5	6	All
Desired Parity:								
x̄	4.56	4.74	4.09	5.81	4.65	3.86	3.57	3.69
SD	2.87	3.22	2.52	3.87	3.07	2.06	1.82	1.92
N	127	113	111	54	405	106	143	249
Child Mortality Rate:								
x̄	17	23	17	20	19	13	15	14
SD	22	23	22	21	22	19	20	20
N	172	167	137	102	578	114	153	269
Female Schooling[1]:								
x̄	1.27	1.03	1.09	.87	1.09	2.87	2.75	2.80
SD	1.56	1.51	1.54	1.18	1.48	3.11	2.42	2.73
N	160	155	128	100	543	110	150	260
Female Literacy:								
Literate	31%	23%	24%	15%	24%	57%	59%	58%
N	50/162	36/158	31/128	15/100	132/548	63/110	89/151	152/261
Male Schooling[1]:								
x̄	1.18	1.13	2.05	.75	1.28	3.70	3.82	3.77
SD	1.74	1.57	1.94	1.25	1.71	3.39	2.85	3.10
N	119	126	95	84	424	102	125	227
Male Literacy:								
Literate	39%	39%	53%	28%	40%	76%	78%	77%
N	52/133	54/139	54/102	25/90	185/464	81/106	98/126	179/232

Table 6-1 (Continued)

	Rural Village (Number)					Semi-urban Community (Number)		
	1	2	3	4	All	5	6	All
Income per Capita (1974–75):								
x̄	110	130	95	82	107	251	180	210
SD	106	135	119	78	115	191	148	171
N	145	148	124	93	510	108	146	254
Land-ownership (cuerdas):								
x̄	57	50	10	64	45	.76	2.51	1.76
SD	123	99	29	101	97	5	9	8
N	147	150	126	94	517	112	150	262
Household Economic Production Type %[2]:								
1	26	18	30	13	22	96	72	82
2	25	18	23	37	25	2	12	8
3	27	28	12	29	24	1	13	8
4	22	35	34	19	28	1	2	2
Female paid labor hours 1975–76:								
x̄	334	547	1352	327	635	868	751	800
SD	949	1116	968	918	1077	1367	1214	1279
N	172	167	137	102	578	112	154	266

[1] Number of grades of schooling completed.
[2] 1 = wage labor; 2 = subsistence farmer; 3 = semi-commercial farmer; and 4 = commercial farmer.

Table 6-1 displays mean values of selected demographic and so-cioeconomic variables describing the sample used in this study. Average female age in the rural sample is 37 years, while it is 34 years in the semi-urban sample. Males average 41 years in the rural, and 39 in the semi-urban sample. Average number of children-ever-born is 5.72 in the rural, and 4.64 in the semi-urban sample. Figures for completed parity are 8.62 and 7.00 for rural and semi-urban, respectively. Child mortality rate is 19 percent in the rural and 14 percent in the semi-urban sample.

Only about one fourth of the rural female respondents are literate, compared with over half the semi-urban females. In both samples literacy figures are higher for males—40 percent in the rural, and 77 percent in the semi-urban, sample. In both samples the average number of grades of schooling completed is low for all: 1.09 for females, and 1.28 for males in the rural; 2.80 for females, and 3.77 for males in the semi-urban sample.

Variables

The main exogenous and endogenous variables are briefly described below:

Female age, measured as a continuous variable, is used as a control for the effect of age on the endogenous variables. Since data on duration of union are unavailable, female age is used as a proxy for exposure to pregnancy, in relation to fertility.

Urbanization is measured as a dichotomy denoting rural versus semi-urban residence.

Child mortality is measured in terms of the proportion of children born that have died, as compared with the total number of live births. The data do not allow specification of infant (as distinct from child) mortality.

Female and male education is measured in terms of literacy. Literacy is a self-report about whether the subject reads and writes well, a little, or not at all. It is used as a dichotomy where zero is assigned to the two first answer-categories (reads and writes a little or not at all) and one to the last category (reads and writes well).

Income is defined as per capita income derived from household total income. Household total income is the sum of (1) total agricultural production in average 1974 prices; (2) total salaries and wages earned by all household members in 1974; and (3) net income earned by all household members from activities in 1974. Unit of measurement is a quetzal (1 quetzal = $1).

Land-ownership means total land owned by the nuclear (and extended) family. Unit of measurement is a *cuerda* (1 *cuerda* = .044 hectares).

Female labor-force participation is measured in terms of total hours worked for pay during 1975–1976—for paid female work only; thus, it measures the degree to which a female is engaged in wage work.

Family type is measured as the number of nuclear families sharing the same house. It thus measures the territorial aspect of family type but excludes the functional aspect (that is, families living apart but sharing income).

Type of economic production is measured as a categorical variable: (1) wage-laborer, (2) subsistence farmer, (3) semi-commercial farmer, and (4) commercial farmer. A family is defined as "wage-laborer" if it reports no agricultural production, but derives its total income from salaries, wages, and nonagricultural activities. Subsistence farmer includes some agricultural production; families in this category sell none of the produce but do hire labor. The semi-commercial farmer family sells some of its agricultural production but does not hire labor. Commercial farmer families do both—sell agricultural production and hire labor.

Family-planning knowledge, attitudes, and practice (KAP) is measured as a simple additive scale: (a) whether the respondent thinks that women ought to have all children that come, or should do something to limit the number; (b) knowledge of a specific way to limit the number of children—coded as (0) no knowledge, (1) knowledge of a "traditional" method, and (2) knowledge of a "modern" method ("traditional" = herbs, rhythm, lactation, withdrawal; "modern" = pill, condom, diaphragm, and/or going to family-planning clinic); and (c) whether respondent does or does not practice a method. The scale ranges from 0 to 4; 0 indicates a position of low pro-family planning and 4, higher pro-family planning.

This family-planning KAP scale measures the respondent's overall family planning position, but not the intensity of family-planning KAP within "traditional" and "modern" dimensions.

Male/female communication is measured as a simple additive scale of four items. Two are the female respondent's report on whether she had (a) talked and (b) agreed with spouse about the number of children desired; the other two are comparisons of (c) male and (d) female respondents' answers to a question about how many additional children they want. This scale ranges from 0 to 4 with 0 indicating low, and 4 higher, male/female communication.

This scale focuses on one aspect of intra-couple communication—namely, the family-size preference, family-planning aspect.

Perceived child utility is measured by means of questionnaire items on female respondent's perceptions both about her children's utility in general and as old-age security. The basic idea is to count how many times the respondent mentions children during the interview. This scale is adapted from a similar scale developed by Eva Mueller (1972). The assumption here is that respondents who mention children as useful in several different contexts (and questionnaire items) are women who perceive and desire greater "utility" from children than do respondents who mention children fewer times or not at all.

The child utility scale, derived from ten items, ranges from 0 to 10 in value, with 0 indicating a low and 10 a higher-perceived utility.

Fertility is measured as the total number of children-ever-born.

Results

Tables 6-2 through 6-4 display results of the empirical analyses. Table 6-2 shows mean and standard deviation of variables. Table 6-3 presents estimated OLS coefficients using the methodology of structural equation model estimation. Table 6-4 displays OLS coefficients from a reduced form equation—that is, estimation of certain direct effects on fertility. Figures 6-1 and 6-2 give the results of Table 6-2 in the form of a path diagram. Estimated coefficients here are reported in both unstandardized and standardized form. Unstandardized coefficients give the change in the dependent variable for a one unit change in the predictor variable. Standardized coefficients yield the expected number of sample standard deviations-change in the dependent variable that would be expected from one standard deviation change in a given predictor variable.

The significant results can be briefly summarized as follows.

Literacy and Fertility

We found female literacy to have a fertility-reducing effect in both the rural and the semi-urban samples. Our results indicate that—

Table 6-2 Mean and Standard Deviation of Variables in Children-Ever-Born Model (Literacy as the Measure of Education)

	Rural (N = 308)		Semi-Urban (N = 91)	
	$\bar{x}$	SD	$\bar{x}$	SD
Age of Female	34	10	35	13
Literacy of Female	.25	.43	.58	.49
Income per Capita	115	140	237	183
Land Ownership	50	100	2	9
Female Paid Labor (hrs.)	535	1025	612	1192
Family Type	1.29	.53	1.33	.65
Parity (children-ever-born)	5.90	3.35	4.92	2.56
Family Planning KAP	1.43	1.36	2.80	1.33
Male/Female Communication	1.88	1.13	2.49	1.20
Perceived Child Utility	3.35	2.21	3.13	2.13
Child Mortality	18	20	16	19
Village Dummy 1	.26	.44	—	—
Village Dummy 2	.32	.47	—	—
Village Dummy 3	.19	.39	—	—
Village Dummy 4	—	—	.38	.49
Literacy of Male	.40	.74	.74	.44

even in the relatively isolated *rural* communities in which the average level of schooling of adults is only one or two years of primary education—being literate does affect one's fertility attitudes and behavior (controlling for other variables) so as to create an incentive for smaller family size.

We would like to note that, in the rural sample, the fertility-reducing effect of female literacy is direct—that is, the effect of literacy on fertility does not operate through the three intervening variables (family planning KAP, male/female communication, and perceived child utility) included in our model (Figure 6-1). This means that in our analyses female literacy influences fertility through intervening variables *not* included in the model. An example of an intervening variable not explicitly included in our model is a mother's aspirations and expectations for her child's schooling and future employment. It is likely that parents' aspirations for children increase with parental educational attainment (Wright, 1965; Shortlidge, n.d.). It is likely also that a mother with greater aspirations for her children's schooling perceives greater costs of child-rearing and therefore has fewer children (Becker and Lewis, 1973; DeTray, 1973; Simon, 1974; Holsinger and Kasada, 1976).

Table 6-3 OLS Coefficients: Literacy as the Measure of Education, Children-Ever-Born Model (T-Statistics in Parentheses)

	Parity Equation				Perceived Child Utility Equation			
	Rural		Semi-Urban		Rural		Semi-Urban	
	b	beta	b	beta	b	beta	b	beta
Age of Female	.561** (7.30)	1.62	.522** (5.84)	2.71	.043** (3.26)	.187	.065** (3.74)	.410
Age of Female Squared	-.005** (-4.70)	-1.07	-.005** (-4.91)	-2.38	—	—	—	—
Literacy of Female	-.740** (-2.52)	-.096	-.566 (-1.39)	-.109	-.056 (-.20)	-.011	-1.40** (-3.16)	-.325
Land	-.009** (-3.22)	-.262	.037 (.36)	.126	-.003* (2.29)	-.129	-.045 (1.65)	-.187
Land Squared	-.000* (-2.38)	-.185	.000 (.04)	.013	—	—	—	—
Income per Capita	—	—	—	—	-.003** (-2.65)	-.151	-.002 (-1.66)	-.172
Female Labor Force Participation	—	—	—	—	.000 (.88)	.053	-.000 (-.86)	-.086
Family Type	—	—	—	—	-.405 (-.177)	-.097	-.401 (-1.23)	-.122
Village Dummy 1	-.351 (-.93)	-.046	—	—	.666 (1.91)	.133	—	—
Village Dummy 2	-.069 (-.19)	-.009	—	—	1.36** (4.08)	.289	—	—
Village Dummy 3	-.262 (.63)	-.031	—	—	.978* (2.41)	.173	—	—
Village Dummy 4	—	—	-.587 (-1.49)	-.119	—	—	.029 (.07)	.007
Family Planning KAP	.053 (.50)	.021	-.139 (-.75)	-.072	—	—	—	—

* $p \leq .05$ ** $p \leq .01$

Table 6-3 (Continued)

	Parity Equation				Perceived Child Utility Equation			
	Rural		Semi-Urban		Rural		Semi-Urban	
	b	beta	b	beta	b	beta	b	beta
Male/Female Communication	-.209 (-1.70)	-.070	.057 (.30)	.026	—	—	—	—
Child Utility	.180** (2.94)	.119	.318** (3.28)	.264	—	—	—	—
Child Mortality	.026** (3.74)	.155	.007 (.76)	.056	—	—	—	—
Constant	-7.50** (-5.66)	—	-6.47** (-3.55)	—	2.01** (3.28)	—	2.84** (3.32)	—
R²	.58		.61		.12		.28	
R² adjusted	.57		.56		.09		.22	
SSE	1433		229		1316		294	
DF	295		80		298		83	
N	308		91		308		91	

	Male/Female Communication Equation				Family Planning KAP Equation			
	Rural		Semi-Urban		Rural		Semi-Urban	
	b	beta	b	beta	b	beta	b	beta
Age of Female	-.004 (-.55)	-.032	-.045** (-4.33)	-.501	-.032** (-4.04)	-.229	-.045** (-4.31)	-.453
Age of Female Squared	—		—		—		—	
Literacy of Female	.055 (.37)	.021	.272 (1.06)	.113	.233 (1.36)	.074	.583* (2.02)	.199

	Coef.	β	Coef.	β	Coef.	β	Coef.	β
Land	−.001 (−.98)	−.057	.019 (1.17)	.138	.001 (1.45)	.083	.001 (.59)	.063
Land Squared	—	—	—	—	—	—	—	—
Income per Capita	.002* (2.38)	.138	−.004* (−2.04)	−.638	.001** (2.58)	.146	−.000 (−.67)	−.066
Female Labor Force Participation	.000 (1.19)	.074	.001 (1.87)	.192	.000 (.68)	.040	−.000 (−.93)	−.090
Family Type	.153 (1.27)	.072	.235 (1.25)	.128	—	—	—	—
Village Dummy 1	−1.49 (−.78)	−.055	—	—	−.156 (−.73)	−.050	—	—
Village Dummy 2	.190 (1.08)	.079	—	—	.503** (2.45)	.172	—	—
Village Dummy 3	−.503* (−2.37)	−.175	—	—	.157 (.63)	.045	—	—
Village Dummy 4	—	—	.234 (.96)	.096	—	—	.737** (2.89)	.269
Family Planning KAP	—	—	—	—	—	—	—	—
Male/Female Communication	—	—	—	—	—	—	—	—
Child Utility	—	—	—	—	—	—	—	—
Child Mortality	—	—	—	—	—	—	—	—
Constant	1.72** (5.39)	—	3.97** (6.65)	—	2.06** (6.45)	—	3.96** (9.29)	—
R^2	.08		.26		.13		.33	
R^2 adjusted	.05		.18		.10		.28	
SSE	360		96		498		108	
DF	298		82		299		84	
N	308		91		308		91	

* $p \leq .05$　　** $p \leq .01$

Table 6-4 OLS Coefficients: Reduced Form with Children-Ever-Born as Dependent Variable, Dummy Variables to Control for Effect of Familial Mode of Production[a] (T-statistics in Parentheses)

	Rural				Semi-urban			
	1	2	3	4	1	2	3	4
Age of Female	.503**	.553**	.569**	.564**	.381**	.387**	.389**	.392**
	(12.40)	(13.81)	(14.43)	(14.21)	(8.55)	(8.66)	(8.79)	(8.81)
Age of Female Squared	-.004**	-.005	-.005**	-.005**	-.003**	-.003**	-.003**	-.003**
	(9.22)	(10.49)	(11.02)	(10.78)	(5.85)	(5.82)	(5.98)	(5.92)
Literacy of Female	-.451	-.511	-.553*	-.595*	-1.11**	-1.11**	-1.16**	-1.16**
	(1.63)	(1.79)	(1.95)	(2.09)	(4.48)	(4.43)	(4.68)	(4.63)
Village Dummy 1	-.874	-.985**	-1.06**	-1.06**	—	—	—	—
	(2.52)	(2.78)	(3.00)	(3.01)				
Village Dummy 2	-.153	-.093	-.217	-.244	—	—	—	—
	(.45)	(.26)	(.62)	(.69)				
Village Dummy 3	-1.16**	-1.32**	-1.34**	-1.44**	—	—	—	—
	(3.17)	(3.54)	(3.60)	(3.85)				
Village Dummy 4	—	—	—	—	.045	—	-.040	-.115
					(.17)		(.16)	(.46)
Economic Mode 1	-1.53**	—	—	—	-.669	.453	—	—
	(5.11)				(1.87)	(.97)		

Table 6-4 (continued)

	Rural				Semi-urban			
	1	2	3	4	1	2	3	4
Economic Mode 2	—	.578* (2.07)	—	—	—	.453 (.97)	—	—
Economic Mode 3	—	—	.447 (1.62)	—	—	—	.682 (1.40)	—
Economic Mode 4	—	—	—	.211 (.79)	—	—	—	.178 (.184)
Constant	-5.33** (6.07)	-6.76** (8.00)	-6.97 (8.21)	-6.82** (8.05)	-3.33** (3.32)	-4.07** (4.42)	-4.07** (4.43)	-4.10** (4.44)
R^2	.50	.48	.47	.47	.53	.53	.53	.53
R^2 adjusted	.49	.47	.47	.46	.52	.52	.52	.52
SSE	3222	3363	3374	3389	859	869	865	872
DF	493	493	493	493	241	241	241	241
N	501	501	501	501	247	247	247	247

* $p \leq .05$ ** $p \leq .01$ *** $p \leq .001$

a Each of the four familial production mode variables are entered in equation separately as follows:

1 = wage labor   3 = semi-commercial farmer
2 = subsistence farmer   4 = commercial farmer

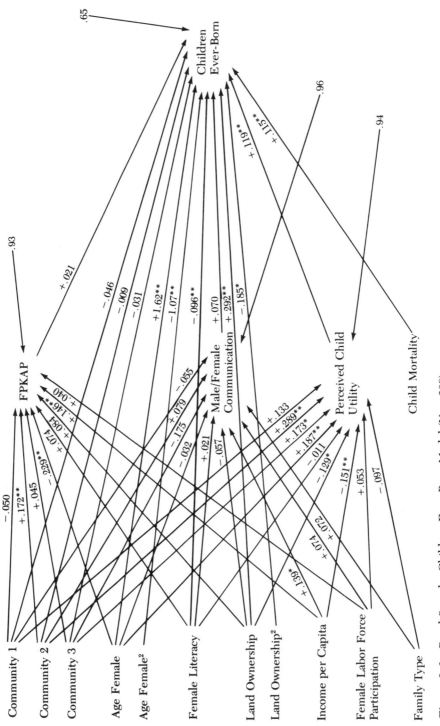

Figure 6-1 Rural Sample: Children Ever-Born Model (N = 308).

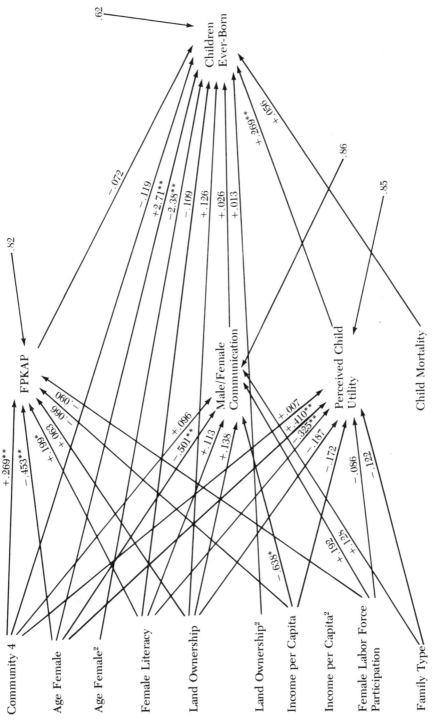

Figure 6-2 Semi-Urban Sample: Children Ever-Born Model (N = 91).

In the semi-urban sample, the fertility-reducing effect of female literacy operates through one of the model's intervening variables: perceived child utility. This may mean that (in the semi-urban context) literacy reduces the perceived material benefits parents expect from children. Also, literate parents, more than illiterate parents, may perceive more costs associated with childbearing. Other empirical studies using urban data from less-developed countries have found a similar, rather strong, effect of education on child utility (Mueller, 1972; Chang, 1976; Mueller and Cohn, 1977).

Income and Fertility

Income per capita is found to have a fertility-reducing effect— operating through perceived child utility—in our rural sample. No effect of income on fertility is observed in the semi-urban sample. In the rural sample, the fertility-reducing effect of income shows that increasing income per capita leads the female head of family to expect less material help from her children (and thus, less need for many offspring). We can argue then that, at least to a certain degree, income substitutes for children in the rural context of LDCs.

Although a controversy exists in the literature about whether income tends to reduce or increase individual fertility in LDCs (Simon, 1974), our finding is similar to what has been noted by some others using LDC data (Mueller, 1972; Mueller and Cohn, 1977). For example, the Value of Children Project (Arnold *et al.*, 1975) has found that the index of expected economic help from children used in that project is in general inversely related to socioeconomic status of family.

Land-Ownership and Fertility

We found that land-ownership has both a direct and indirect effect on fertility in the rural sample, but no effect on fertility in the semi-urban sample.

The direct effect of land-ownership on fertility is curvilinear in our rural sample. In other words, as the family acquires more land (or wealth and resources in general), its fertility increases initially but, after attaining a threshold-level of wealth, fertility starts to decline.

The above finding is very relevant to the existing debate in the fertility-determinants literature on whether land-ownership induces or reduces individual fertility in LDCs (Ajami, 1969 and 1976; de-Janvry, 1976; Stokes *et al.*, 1979). On one hand, some argue that

land-ownership increases fertility; on the other hand, other researchers maintain that land-ownership reduces fertility. Our results
suggest that it is not one or the other, but rather both. Initially,
increases in wealth induce fertility (because of improved fecundity
and enhanced capacity to afford children). In the long run, however,
and when a certain level of wealth has been attained, further increases in wealth tend to reduce fertility.

In our analyses land-ownership is found to have an indirect
fertility-reducing effect, operating through perceived child utility;
this is in addition to the observed direct fertility effect in the rural
sample. Thus it seems that land-ownership, like per capita income,
tends to be a substitute for children in representing general social
and old-age security for rural areas of LDCs. This is to be expected
since, in many ways, land-ownership seems to be a more reliable
source of general social and old-age security than are children; after
all, children die, move away, and may not be willing nor able to
support parents.

Mode of Familial Production and Fertility

Prior to the analyses presented in the tables of this chapter, some
cross-tabulations showed that wage-laborer families have consistently lower parities and perceived child utility than do the different
categories of farmers, in both our rural and semi-urban samples. For
example, in the rural sample, average number of children-ever-born
at completed parity (for women aged 45–55) is 7.4 for wage-laborer
families, 8.7 for subsistence farmer families, 9.2 for semi-commercial
farmer families, and 8.3 for commercial farmer families.

In order to assess the effect on fertility of mode of familial production, while controlling the effects of other variables on fertility, OLS
regression analyses were undertaken. An example of these results is
displayed in Table 6-3. Note that in an effort to control for multicollinearity, the reduced-form equations are reestimated with each
production dummy variable in the equation, one at a time. Table 6-3
shows that mode of familial production affects fertility in both rural
and semi-urban samples: For both samples, belonging to a wage-
labor family has a fertility-reducing effect, whereas belonging to one
of the farmer categories tends to increase fertility. This is an important result, since not much is known about how and why individual
demographic behavior varies by mode-of-production groups (Ajami,
1969; Mueller and Cohen, 1977).

Our results suggest that, in both the rural and semi-urban context, if a family derives its income from wages rather than from selling produce, then on the average that family tends to have fewer children. The most common way to explain the lower fertility of wage-laborer families is by comparing the lesser reliance on children as labor sources by wage-laborer families, with the greater need of farmers for as many hands as possible to carry out the many labor-intensive farm tasks (Mamdani, 1972; White, 1976; Folbre, 1976; Nag, Peete, and White, 1978).

Other Variables and Fertility

In addition to the observed effects on fertility of female literacy, family economic production, and perceptions of child utility, we found that certain other variables showed a consistent effect on fertility. These variables are: female age, community of residence of the individual family, and child mortality.

The strong association between female age and fertility is expected, reflecting as it does the importance of life cycle. Residence in a particular community affects fertility through perceptions of child utility; residence in (rural) Villages 2 and 3, for example, increases perceived child utility. It is interesting to note that these two communities differ from the other rural villages in that an income-generating activity is available in Villages 2 and 3 which requires a large quantity of labor but relatively little physical strength—that is, an activity easily performed by children. We suspect that the availability of income-generating activities for children in the community at large increases parents' perceptions of child utility and, subsequently, affects fertility.

And last, we would like to note the relatively strong association in our rural sample between child mortality and fertility. This result coincides with a large body of evidence suggesting that parents in LDCs choose to have several children partially to replace those who may die, and also to insure that a certain number will survive to support the parents in old age (Schultz, 1976; Preston, 1978).

In summary, we found that the most consistent, significant factors affecting individual fertility are female literacy, family economic production characteristics, and the female head of family's perceptions about child utility. Note that, of the intervening variables considered in this study (family-planning KAP, male/female communication, and perceived child utility), only perceived child utility shows an effect on fertility. In terms of *total* effects (adding direct and indirect effects), in the rural-area, mode of production—that is, to belong to a wage-laborer family—produces the largest fertility-reducing effect. Of the socioeconomic variables in the semi-urban area, female literacy shows the largest fertility-reducing effect.

Conclusions

We have reported results from analyses of determinants of fertility using cross-sectional household survey data from four rural and two semi-urban Ladino communities in Guatemala. The focus has been on the role of education of female head of household and familial economic production on number of children-ever-born. We have looked at the effects on fertility of education and familial economic production in the context of a path model of socioeconomic and attitudinal variables and fertility.

The most consistent factors that affected fertility at the level of the individual family were found, in the *rural* sample, to be female literacy, family economic production, and· female head of family's perceptions of child utility. In the *semi-urban* sample those factors were female literacy and perceptions of child utility.

It would appear from our analyses that families in LDCs have many children—mainly for socioeconomic reasons, and because children are perceived as a means of production and protection. Our results suggest (as has been suggested elsewhere in the fertility-determinants literature: see Mamdani, 1972; Caldwell, 1976; Folbre, 1976; Wolfson, 1978) that the relatively high fertility found in LDCs is in large part economically rational behavior, given the context and alternatives available to the majority of families in these countries.

That we find female literacy to have a fertility-reducing effect controlling for socioeconomic status is important, for it suggests that even when women may appear to have little use for schooling and literacy, literacy in fact does affect the lives of women, and families, in critical ways. Considering that, worldwide and on every continent, the majority of the illiterate are women and that the situation is not really improving (Newland, 1979), there is an urgent need to increase radically efforts and resources for women's schooling, particularly in rural areas of LDCs.

Our results indicate that in the long run the improved socioeconomic condition of the family will contribute significantly to a de-

crease in fertility. These results accentuate the importance of indirect (rather than direct) population policies. Direct policies—that is,
family-planning programs—do have a role to play in population
policy, but only in connection with indirect policies such as the
following:

1. Improving access of females to schooling and literacy.
2. Providing parents with ways of maintaining or increasing
    production that do not depend on children's work. Such mea-
    sures as, for example, increases in wages and in the capacity
    of small-scale farmers to become more productive and to sell
    at better prices will make it less necessary for lower-income
    wage-laborers and farmers to rely on children for production
    of goods for supplementary consumption, within the house-
    hold and for exchange (to be sold in the market).
3. Providing parents with alternative sources of security, other
    than children, (a) by reducing the high degree of insecurity of
    disadvantaged groups in LDCs and (b) by improving access to
    different forms of social security: for unemployment, health,
    and old age.
4. Improving female status in traditionally feminine roles and
    providing alternatives to those existing roles. The purpose is
    to facilitate women's daily production activities within and
    outside the household, and to increase women's control over
    the income/wealth that women generate (Dixon, 1978).

Ultimately, the purpose of population policy ought to be to promote women's and men's capacity to control their own lives better
and to choose when and whether to bear children. Providing knowledge and access to contraception is not the only answer; it will take a
combination of measures designed to improve women's status, the
socioeconomic condition of the family, and to provide family planning in the context of family health care (Tabarrah, 1971;
McGreevey and Birdsall, 1974; Wolfson, 1978).

References

AJAMI, I. "Social Class, Family Demographic Characteristics and Mobility in Three
    Iranian Villages." *Sociologia Ruralis 9*, 1969.
AJAMI, I. "Differential Fertility in Peasant Communities: A Study of Six Iranian
    Villages." *Population Studies 30*, 1976.

ARNOLD, F. *et al. The Value of Children: A Cross-National Study.* Honolulu: East-West Population Institute, East-West Center, 1975.

BAGOZZI, R. P., and M. F. VAN LOO. "Toward a General Theory of Fertility: A Causal Modeling Approach." *Demography*, August, 1978.

BECKER, G., and H. G. LEWIS. "On the Interaction between Quantity and Quality of Children." *Journal of Political Economy 81*, 2, Part II (March/April 1973).

BERELSON, B. *Family Planning and Population Programs.* A Review of World Developments. Chicago: University of Chicago Press, 1966.

BINDARY, A. *et al.* "Urban-Rural Differences in the Relationship Between Women's Employment and Fertility: A Preliminary Study." *Journal of Biosocial Science 5*, 2 (April 1973).

CALDWELL, J. "Toward a Restatement of Demographic Transition Theory." *Population and Development Review 2*, 3 and 4 (September/December 1976).

CARVAJAL, M. J., and D. T. GEITHMAN. *Family Planning and Family Size Determination.* The Evidence from Seven Latin American Cities. Gainesville: University Presses of Florida, 1976.

CASSEN, R. H. "Population and Development: A Review." *World Development 4* (October 11, 1976).

CELADE and CFSC. *Fertility and Family Planning in Metropolitan Latin America.* Chicago: Community and Fertility Study Center, University of Chicago, 1972.

CHANG, L. T. "Desired Fertility, Income and the Valuation of Children." ILO, Population and Employment Working Paper, No. 36, March 1976.

CICRED. *Seminar on Infant Mortality in Relation to the Level of Fertility.* Conference report. Bangkok, 1976.

COCHRANE, S. *Education and Fertility: What Do We Really Know.* Washington, D.C.: World Bank, 1978.

DAVIDSON, M. "Female Work Status and Fertility in Latin America." In *The Fertility of Working Women*, edited by S. Kupinsky. New York: Praeger, 1977.

DAVIS, K. "Institutional Patterns Favoring High Fertility in Underdeveloped Areas." *Eugenics Quarterly 2*, 1955.

DEERE, C. D., and A. DEJANVRY. "A Conceptual Framework for the Empirical Analysis of Peasants." Giannini Foundation of Agricultural Economics, Division of Agricultural Sciences, University of California, Berkeley, December 1978.

DE JANVRY, A. "The Political Economy of Rural Development in Latin America: An Interpretation: Reply." *American Journal of Agricultural Economics 58*, 1976.

DE TRAY, D. N. *An Economic Analysis of Quantity-Quality Substitution in Household Fertility Decisions.* Santa Monica, California: RAND Corporation, 1973, P-4449.

DIXON, R. *Rural Women at Work.* Baltimore: The Johns Hopkins University Press, 1978.

DUNCAN, O. D. *Introduction to Structural Equation Models.* New York: Academic Press, 1975.

FOLBRE, N. "Economics and Population Control." *Science for the People 8* (November-December 1976).

GOLDSTEIN, S. "The Influence of Labor Force Participation and Education on Fertility in Thailand." *Population Studies 26*, 3 (November 1972).

HILL, R. *et al.* "Intra-Family Communication and Fertility in Puerto Rico." *Rural Sociology XX* (September/December 1955).

HOFFMAN, L. W., and M. L. HOFFMAN. "The Value of Children to Parents." In *Psychological Perspectives on Population*, edited by J. T. Fawcett. New York: Basic Books, 1973.

HOLSINGER, D. B., and J. D. KASADA. "Education and Fertility: Sociological Perspectives." In *Population and Development*, edited by R. G. Ridker. Baltimore: The Johns Hopkins University Press, 1976.

LEIBENSTEIN, H. *Economic Backwardness and Economic Growth.* New York: John Wiley & Sons, 1957.

MACFARLANE, A. "Modes of Reproduction." *Journal of Development Studies 14*, 4 (July 1978).

MAMDANI, M. *The Myth of Population Control: Family, Caste and Class in an Indian Village.* New York: Monthly Review Press, 1972.

McGREEVEY, W. P., and N. BIRDSALL. *The Policy Relevance of Recent Social Research on Fertility.* Washington, D.C.: Smithsonian Institution, 1974.

MEJIA PIVARAL, V. "Caracteristicas Economicas y Socioculturales de Cuatro Aldeas Ladinas de Guatemala." *Guatemala Indigena VII*, 3, 1972.

MUELLER, E. "Economic Motives for Family Limitation: A Study Conducted in Taiwan." *Population Studies 26*, 3 (November 1972).

MUELLER, E., and R. COHN. "The Relation of Income to Fertility Decisions in Taiwan." *Economic Development and Cultural Change 25*, 2 (January 1977).

NAG, M., C. PEETE, and B. WHITE. "An Anthropological Approach to the Study of the Economic Value of Children in Java and Nepal." *Current Anthropology 19*, 2 (June 1978).

NAMBOODIRI, N. K. "Some Observations on the Economic Framework for Fertility Analysis." *Population Studies 26* (July 1972).

NAMBOODIRI, N. K. "Which Couples at Given Parities Expect to Have Additional Births? An Exercise in Discriminant Analysis." *Demography 11*, 1974.

NEWLAND, K. *The Sisterhood of Man.* New York: Norton Company, 1979.

PRESTON, S. *The Effects of Infant and Child Mortality on Fertility.* New York: Academic Press, 1978.

SCHULTZ, T. P. "An Economic Model of Family Planning and Fertility." *Journal of Political Economy 77*, 2 (March/April 1969).

SCHULTZ, T. P. "Interrelationships Between Mortality and Fertility." In *Population and Development*, edited by R. G. Ridker. Baltimore: The Johns Hopkins University Press, 1976.

SEAR, A. M. "Predictors of Contraceptive Practice for Low Income Women in Cali, Colombia." *Journal of Biosocial Science 7* (1975): 171–188.

SHORTLIDGE, R. L. "A Socioeconomic Model of School Attendance in Rural India." Center for Human Resource Research, Ohio State University.

SIMON, J. L. *The Effects of Income on Fertility.* Chapel Hill, N.C.: Carolina Population Center, University of North Carolina, 1974.

SIMON, J. L. "Income, Wealth, and Their Distribution." In *Population and Development*, edited by R. G. Ridker. Baltimore: The Johns Hopkins University Press, 1976.

SIMONEN, M. "Education, Production and Fertility: The Case of Rural and Semi-Urban Ladino Guatemala." Unpublished Ph.D. dissertation. University of California, Berkeley, July 1980.

STOKES, C. S. *et al.* "Rural Development, Land, and Human Fertility: A State-of-the-Arts Paper." Durham, North Carolina: Research Triangle Institute, 1979.

TABBARAH, R. B. 1971. "Toward a Theory of Demographic Development." *Economic Development and Cultural Change 19*, 2 (January 1971).

WHITE, B. "Production and Reproduction in a Javanese Village." Unpublished Ph.D. dissertation. New York: Columbia University, 1976.

WILLIAMS, A. D. "Determinants of Fertility in Developing Countries—Review and Evaluation of Literature." In *Population, Public Policy and Economic Development*, edited by M. C. Keeley. New York: Praeger Press, 1976.

WOLFSON, M. *Changing Approaches to Population Problems*. Paris: Development Centre, OECD, 1978.

WRIGHT, P. C. *The Role and Effects of Literacy in a Guatemalan Ladino Peasant Community*. Tampa: University of South Florida, 1965.

WYON, J. B., and GORDON, J. E. *The Khana Study: Population Problems in the Rural Punjab*. Cambridge, Mass.: Harvard University Press, 1971.

TECHNICAL APPENDIX

The model in Figure 6.2 can be written out as the following set of structural equations:

$$X_{11i} = \alpha_{11} + \beta_{111}X_{1i} + \beta_{112}X_{2i} + \beta_{114}X_{4i} + \beta_{115}X_{5i} + \beta_{117}X_{7i} + \beta_{119}X_{9i}$$
$$+ \; \epsilon_{11i}$$

$$X_{12i} = \alpha_{12} + \beta_{121}X_{1i} + \beta_{122}X_{2i} + \beta_{124}X_{4i} + \beta_{125}X_{5i} + \beta_{127}X_{7i} + \beta_{128}X_{8i}$$
$$+ \; \beta_{129}X_{9i} + \beta_{1210}X_{10i} + \epsilon_{12i}$$

$$X_{13i} = \alpha_{13} + \beta_{131}X_{1i} + \beta_{132}X_{2i} + \beta_{134}X_{4i} + \beta_{135}X_{5i} + \beta_{137}X_{7i} + \beta_{139}X_{9i}$$
$$+ \; \beta_{1310}X_{10i} + \epsilon_{13i}$$

$$X_{15i} = \alpha_{15} + \beta_{151}X_{1i} + \beta_{152}X_{2i} + \beta_{153}X_{3i} + \beta_{154}X_{4i} + \beta_{155}X_{5i} + \beta_{156}X_{6i}$$
$$+ \; \beta_{1511}X_{11i} + \beta_{1512}X_{12i} + \beta_{1513}X_{13i} + \beta_{1514}X_{14i} + \epsilon_{15}$$

Chapter 7

SYNTHESIS OF FINDINGS AND POLICY IMPLICATIONS

by Judith B. Balderston

Chapter 1 began with the theme that, for better planning, we need more knowledge about several aspects of rural poverty. We suggested that research could disentangle relationships among the conditions of poor health, poor diet, illiteracy, overcrowding, and low productivity that characterize the lives of many in poor rural communities throughout the world. We discussed the need for investigation, separately within biological, social, and economic areas, and also where they intersect. Such understanding, we suggested, could help planners and policy-makers in choosing how to allocate resources.

In this final chapter we want to summarize the most important findings from the Berkeley group's analysis of data collected in the Guatemala experiment—the subjects of Chapters 3 to 6. By drawing together results of these four sub-studies we show interrelationships among the parts as each affects the well-being of children and families. We shall discuss methods of intervention to improve well-being and suggest an ordering of interventions and an intergenerational time table.

Information from such a microstudy, of course, is only one component of policy-making. Specific policy interventions depend on assessing institutional conditions and human needs, on the costs of alternatives, on agreement on goals and objectives, on the role of government responsibility, and on the preferences of decision-makers. Policy interventions in any one particular case should depend also on the resource base of that society and on the degree of urgency for development. Although studies such as ours are useful

177

in helping people choose which decision may be made, actual decisions and implementations are subject to a variety of economic and political factors.

We also recognize that, although we have dealt solely with a study conducted in Guatemala, the results, in part, can be generalized to other, similar environments. Biological relationships appear to be of a general nature while economic, social, and cultural factors tend to be specific to their environment. Translation of our results to any other setting would require knowledge of conditions within that setting.

In spite of these constraints, we feel obliged, as careful observers of the extensive and lengthy experiment and data collection in Guatemala, to discuss the policy implications of our findings at the micropolicy level. Extension of our results to the macrolevel or to the dynamics of the longer run necessarily would have to be the subject of other work.

Programs may be conceived in response to one or a combination of several goals—increasing productivity and economic development, providing basic needs for the poorest members of society, redistributing income, equalizing opportunity—and these programs may take the form of single or multiple interventions. Recent work in the international development field emphasizes the need for integrated planning to achieve multiple goals. The World Bank (1975, 1980) has consistently argued that interventions be integrated for greater efficiency. Much recent work in nutrition and health planning, demography, economics, and rural development has asserted that effective decision-making requires multisectoral planning.

Linkages between nutrition, health, and population (Winikoff and Brown, 1980), the role of health in development (Grosse and Harkany, 1980), and health in the assault on poverty (McEvers, 1980) have been the subject of recent reviews. In the demography literature (Leibenstein, 1974; and Easterlin, 1977) a recurrent theme has been the recognition that, if family planning is to be accepted, change must take place in the basic economic conditions of the family as well as in the survival rate of children. The Narangawal population study in India (C. E. Taylor *et al.*, 1975) has shown that receptivity to family planning is greater when family-planning promotion occurs in conjunction with nutrition and health interventions. Nutrition planners (see, for example, Berg and Muscat, 1973) have argued for a systems approach, recognizing that nutrition is connected to many other sectors in a complex set of relationships.

Education-planning linkages to nutrition have been explored only recently (see Mushkin, 1979).

But integrated planning is fraught with difficulty. Johnston (1977), reviewing the pursuit of multiple objectives in food, health, and population planning, discusses how hard it is to achieve integrated planning and resource allocation because objectives, means, and constraints are so interrelated and sometimes conflicting. To design strategies means making hard choices; resources are limited and consensus about public priorities is difficult to achieve. In nutrition and family planning, for example, numerous interventions were failures—and these failures disillusioned many decision-makers.

When planning demands coordination among several sectors, even greater difficulty arises. Johnston recommends the careful study of alternatives through evaluating field interventions and reviewing the experimental evidence accumulated in microstudies. (See also Johnston and Meyer, 1977.) Johnston cautions that, because of the large number of interacting variables, clear-cut answers are not always available. He recommends involving social scientists with planners in all the separate planning sectors.

Recognizing that it is theoretically desirable to integrate programs has, thus far, had very little influence on the behavior of bureaucracies. It is hard to think of situations in which bureaucrats voluntarily have shared budgets with other sectors. While schools do offer lunch programs—shown to be of limited nutritional consequence (Reed, 1973)—preschool nutrition or health programs which could significantly affect subsequent school performance have never been recommended by education planners. It has become more popular to push for joint rural development and nonformal education programs; rarely, however, has the contribution of education to agricultural efficiency been stressed outside academic literature. Health ministries almost never address malnutrition problems, preferring to concentrate on providing health-care facilities. Since bureaucrats are seldom rewarded for efforts that cross sectoral lines or require long time-horizons, it appears difficult indeed to try restructuring bureaucracies and their methods of allocating resources, in the light of multiple objectives.

Moreover, unresolved arguments remain: What is properly of public concern, and what should be left to the consumer and the private sector? When resources are scarce, as they almost always are, governments are unlikely to take on additional areas of public responsibility. Sectors such as education and health traditionally are public while others, such as nutrition and family planning, are left to individual choice and the consumer's ability to pay.

In sum, bureaucracies that want to initiate plans in response to multiple goals will have to agree on objectives and on methods of allocating resources. Understanding the value of trade-offs between areas—how response to one program might affect outcomes in another—must become an important part of the decision process in increasing the effectiveness and efficiency of programs. It is to increase this knowledge that our results are presented.

Research Results of the Berkeley Study

In this section we summarize findings of the Berkeley Project on Education and Nutrition, identifying linkages between parts of our study and pointing to those results that may be most significant for policy purposes. Because of the wide range of data collected by INCAP and RAND on families and individual children in the four villages, we have been able to go beyond the questions that originally engaged us—of nutritional effects on school performance—to investigate relationships that connect nutrition, schooling, work, family size, and agricultural production. Analytical results obtained from these investigations make it possible for us to integrate our findings, providing information necessary for formulating consistent policies.

Chapters 3 through 6 present four related but separate studies that used information that INCAP and RAND collected in the four villages. The most important results will be summarized in this chapter. Each set of statistically significant findings, we believe, is important and robust, for both research and planning.

In addition to the separate findings of each of the studies (the longitudinal models on child nutrition and growth; and the three cross-sectional models on schooling and work, literacy and agricultural efficiency, and literacy and fertility), we suggest that results of the four studies can be viewed as an integrated whole. The studies are related not only because all are based on the same four villages, but also because the variables themselves measure conditions that are interrelated in the lives of the villagers.

We must caution that, although we shall seek to integrate the findings, we did not combine variables from the four parts of the analysis into one complete and comprehensive model. Limitations of time and available computer space precluded this. Besides, constraints imposed by missing data would have made it impossible to construct one intergenerational model that would include a full set of economic, biological, psychological, and educational variables. We relied instead on carrying out separate studies based on sets of data that were similar in important characteristics. Following these separate analyses, we were then able to relate each set of results to the other sets.

Summary of Findings

From the series of estimations using longitudinal models carried out by Alan Wilson in Chapter 3, we have seen that:

1. Supplementation (but not home diet) has a significant effect on growth in weight and height. The most significant supplementation effect was to increase the proportion of diet drawn from protein sources. Protein supplementation shows a strong positive effect on growth, especially up to 48 months. Diarrhea affects annual increments of growth negatively, as do other forms of illness, especially in the Fresco villages.

2. Combining calories and protein from both home diet and both kinds of supplementation shows that there is a significant effect of protein on growth that appears between ages 12 and 36 months. Again we see the consistent negative effect of diarrhea upon growth.

3. A highly significant positive relationship between height and verbal development shows up at all ages. This is the most important result of this section: Taller children do better on verbal tests, controlling for wealth (CONSUMP is a factor score of family possessions). CONSUMP itself is a significant predictor. Verbal test scores are related to sex (girls do better than boys), morbidity, and family structure (children from nuclear families do worse than others); and positively to parental literacy and modernity backgrounds and to family size (especially where there is a higher proportion of older family members at the time of the subject's birth).

4. School enrollment is positively affected by verbal factor scores, by sex, by height, by the number of younger siblings at the time the subject is six, by parental literacy and modernity, and by occupation of mother, but not of father.

5. Verbal factor scores have a highly significant positive effect on teacher-assessments of a child. Concurrent diet has a substantial, and very significant, effect upon teacher-assessments.

6. Among factors that appear most influential on height, weight, and verbal development, there is a strong sequential influence from one period to the next. Such measures show stability from one period to another.

7. Mother's attendance at the supplementation center is a strong determinant of child's intake of supplementation, particularly in the Atole villages.

From cross-sectional analysis carried out by Judith Balderston and presented in Chapter 4, it was seen that:

8. When family's need for the child's work is the same, taller, healthier children are more likely to attend at least a full year of school than are smaller, less healthy children.

9. Children from more affluent farming families work more (and also go to school more) than children of the less affluent. This may be the result of the need for children's work (because of larger landholdings), but also it may show that more vigorous children engage in greater total activity.

10. Earlier-born children are more likely than their younger siblings to attend school. Children of larger families are less likely to attend than children from smaller ones.

11. Parental literacy positively affects school attendance and achievement of children. Parental literacy is positively related also to affluence.

12. The opportunity for children to engage in paid work in commercial cash-crop production is important in determining high participation in the labor market and low participation in school. This is especially evident in Village 2 where, during a several-year period, school participation is relatively low compared to the other villages.

Maria Freire's analysis, presented in Chapter 5, showed that:

13. Literate farmers are more productive than those who are illiterate. Literate farmers use more chemical inputs and raise relatively more cash crops. Even after controlling for chemical inputs and kinds of crops grown, education was a significant factor in explaining variations in output.

14. The impact of education on productivity appeared to differ among farming groups. Literacy made the greatest difference

for the middle range of farmers. For commercial farmers, productivity appeared unaffected by the amount of education.

15. Production of traditional crops appeared to be less affected by literacy of the farmer than was the output of crops for which innovation in planting and fertilizing is of importance.

Mari Simonen's analysis in Chapter 6 showed that:

16. Female literacy was found to have a significant, direct, negative effect on fertility (children-ever-born) while male literacy was found to have no effect.

17. Land ownership (wealth) was found to have a significant, direct, curvilinear (first positive and, after a threshold level, negative) effect on fertility. In addition, both land ownership and income-per-capita were found to have a significant, indirect (through perceived child utility), negative effect on fertility.

18. In the analyses of determinants of fertility, perceived child-utility (that is, the perceived benefits of children in helping parents and providing old-age security) showed a consistent positive effect on fertility.

19. Important differences in the effects on fertility of the variables considered were found to derive from different types of economic production of family. For example, to belong to a semi-commercial familial production unit has a significant, positive effect on fertility (children-ever-born) through perceived child utility, while belonging to the other types of production units produces no such effect.

The strongest and most important conclusions of our analyses are:

(a) Protein supplementation during early childhood has a positive effect on growth. Height, verbal development, and school enrollment, all are affected positively by protein supplementation. Total diet has a strong effect on school achievement. Diarrhea has negative effects on all the same variables.

(b) Children's school enrollment and achievement also are positively affected by parental affluence and by the need for the children's work. Village differences appear to affect patterns of work and school participation differentially. In one village, school participation is consistently low, and affluence of family appears to be the strongest influence, affecting school enrollment positively. In the

other three villages, enrollment is more positively affected by child size and health, and less by family
affluence. Family occupation, sex, and family size also
affect child's activities and school participation.

(c) Schooling of farmers relates positively to agricultural
production. Literate farmers accept innovation more
readily and are able to achieve higher agricultural returns
than illiterate farmers.

(d) Schooling of female heads of household affects the number of children-ever-born, and perceptions of the economic utility of children. It is expected that women will
have fewer children as family economic conditions improve because the perceived utility of children will be
reduced.

From these conclusions, we see from (a) that with improved nutrition and improved health conditions (medical care, potable water,
better sanitation) children will be more likely to attend, and to
achieve in, school. With improved schooling of males (assuming that
the men continue to be farming decision-makers), we see from
(c) that such farmers will achieve higher productivity, increased
affluence, and perceive less need for children's work. Improved
schooling of females will lead, as shown from (d), first to lowered
perceptions of the need for children's help and subsequently to
smaller families. Higher production and lower family size leads to
higher per-capita income and better nutrition for family members.
This in turn makes for the better school performance that results also
from better health, physical and verbal development, and parental
literacy.

We see that education is pivotal. Literacy is one instrument
through which farmers innovate and by which women's attitudes
concerning the economic need for children are affected. Educational
performance depends on children's well-being and on the family's
lessened need for their work. Children with poor health and chronic
malnutrition may never realize their full physical and psychological
potential. To improve chances of success in school, the early health
and nutrition of children should be improved.

We portray our results diagrammatically, which may both confuse
and enlighten; C. W. Churchman (1979, p. 231) calls this the es-
sence of the systems approach. Figure 7-1 presents research results
of the Berkeley project from the perspective of the child's develop-

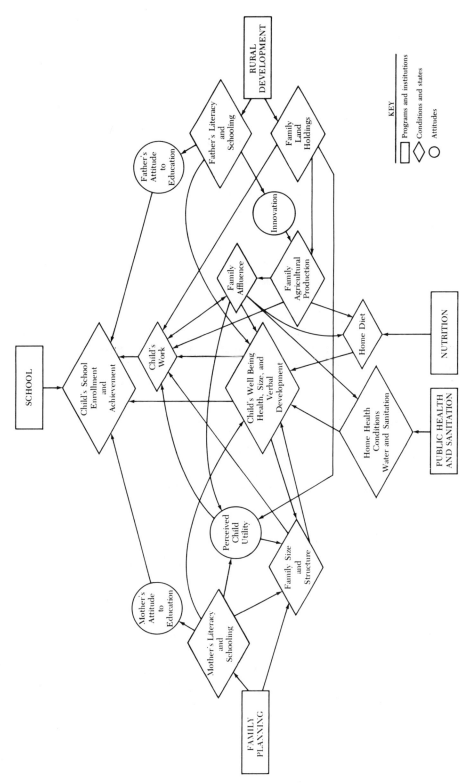

Figure 7-1 Nutrition, Health, Education, Agricultural Production, and Fertility: Interactions Among Sectors from the Perspective of the Child's Development.

ment. The diagram portrays the interaction among interventions, conditions, and perceptions and is intended to show the inter-relationship of family economic conditions, parental literacy, family size, health, diet, school, and work. Relationships center upon the child's well-being, and the outcomes of well-being in terms of school and work. Arrows represent significant and important relationships found in the course of the study in Berkeley.

This diagram, combining results from the four parts of our study, shows that the child's development is affected by family affluence and need to work, family size and structure, nutritional intake, quality of family diet and health conditions, and parental literacy. Improving the child's conditions at an early age leads to inter-generational benefits as that child reaches maturity. At adulthood, men's literacy and schooling appear to influence productivity as farmers; for women, literacy and schooling appear to influence at-titudes about desirable family size. In combination with other devel-opment efforts, then, education can be an effective method for increasing per-capita income through its effects on increasing pro-ductivity and lowering family size.

Program Interventions

The five program interventions which we have discussed can be combined into 31 possible combinations. Figure 7-2 represents these combinations of interventions. By "interventions," we mean the following:

1. *Nutrition:* Direct interventions (such as improvement by supplementation, family food allotments, food stamps, etc.) aimed to reach specific target groups or the whole commu-nity.
2. *Public Health:* Provision of potable water, sanitation, and public health clinics.
3. *Education:* Improved school facilities, classes, and materials; to be added to existing schools.
4. *Rural Development:* Agricultural extension services, loans, and/or provisions of irrigation equipment, fertilizer, and seed.
5. *Family Planning:* Provision of information and methods (pos-sible to be integrated with health-clinic services).

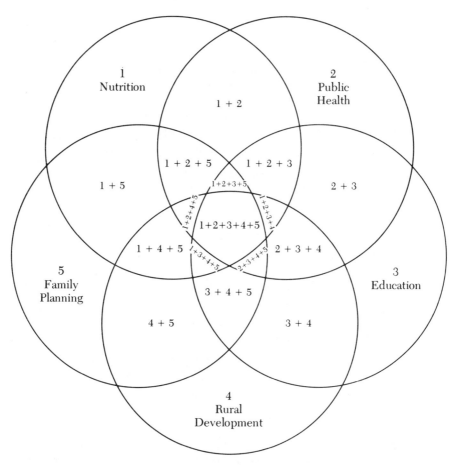

This diagram includes ten additional combinations that could not be portrayed graphically:

1 + 3	1 + 2 + 4
1 + 4	1 + 3 + 4
2 + 4	1 + 3 + 5
2 + 5	2 + 3 + 5
3 + 5	2 + 4 + 5

Figure 7-2   Representation of all Possible Interventions Combining Sectors.

The discussion that follows is based on our research findings. Since a wide range of programs can take place within each type of intervention and because cost will vary with the amount of service provided, it is beyond the scope of this book to suggest the intensity of each intervention.

Intervention	Discussion
1 Nutrition	Nutritional intervention alone (without upgrading general public-health conditions) would benefit only children already relatively free of diarrheal disease. Our results indicate that children's growth is not affected by nutritional intake alone but depends also upon the body's ability to use nutrients. It would be inefficient to undertake this intervention alone.
2 Public Health	Potable water and sanitation reduce the incidence of diarrheal disease. This intervention would reach the poorest children. Over the short run it would be more efficient if combined with a nutritional intervention. Over the long run the resultant decreased infant mortality (leading to larger families) might have adverse effects on per-capita income, unless attempts were made also both to increase income and decrease family size.
3 Education	Investments in education alone, in the absence of improved health and nutritional intake, will tend to benefit children from relatively more affluent families—children already able to attend and profit from schooling.
4 Rural Development	Programs directed at improving agricultural practice appear most beneficial for literate farmers, who tend to accept innovation, and for farmers with access to adequate land. To reach others, increased education through adult literacy programs, plus access to better land, would increase the effectiveness of rural development programs. Rural development alone would not reach the poorest, least-educated people.
5 Family Planning	Family-planning programs seem to influence most the attitudes of women who are literate, and who count less on children for economic utility. To increase the acceptability of family planning, the need for children as a source of labor and security to parents will have to be removed. This intervention alone, then, tends to be relatively inefficient.
1+2 Nutrition and Public Health	A combination of public-health and nutritional interventions would improve the body's use of food intake through lowered incidence of diarrhea and would promote children's health and physical growth. As a

Intervention	Discussion
	result, potential school performance also would benefit. Nutritional supplementation, in the long run, is not desirable because of its high cost and increased family dependency on outside aid. In the short run, nutritional intervention should be given to infants and young children in order to improve their chances of success in school and, consequently, greater productivity as adults.
1+3 Nutrition and Education	Nutritional intervention and increased investment in education are wasteful without public-health intervention, necessary to improve the benefits of food. Increasing expenditures for education would tend to benefit most those already able to attend school.
1+4 Nutrition and Rural Development	Again, improving nutritional intake without health change is wasteful. Rural development intervention alone will tend to benefit those already receptive to innovation—most likely, literate farmers. Besides, since nutritional assistance tends to increase dependence on food relief, while rural-development activities aim to increase independence, combining these activities appears incompatible.
1+5 Nutrition and Family Planning	As before, it is inefficient to improve nutrition without including public-health interventions. Family-planning interventions taken alone also are inefficient because of the low level of acceptability of information, unless accompanied both by change in economic conditions and female literacy.
2+3 Public Health and Education	Better health conditions, sanitation, and potable water would improve the health and physical development of children, making it possible for them to use the family diet more efficiently. Larger, healthier children will do better in school; and increased investment in school also may raise the level of school participation. However, this combination will not meet the needs of the more malnourished children.
2+4 Public Health and Rural Development	Rural development plus public-health services would improve the health and vigor of adults and children while helping farmers adopt more efficient methods. The most malnourished children will not be helped.

Intervention	Discussion
2+5 Public Health and Family Planning	Public health and family planning can be combined in a synergistic delivery system with mutually enhancing benefits. With public health improvements it is expected that more infants will survive, and thus family planning would be directed at discouraging higher family size. However, we found that family-planning information does not tend to influence the attitudes of illiterate women and/or those who perceive children to be useful in work and for old-age security.
3+4 Education and Rural Development	To combine these investments will tend to improve the productivity of families with literate members, and will increase the level of performance of children already able to attend school. It does not reach the poorest families.
3+5 Education and Family Planning	Education and family planning eventually would be mutually beneficial. Education of females would result in more receptivity to family-planning information. Those who remain illiterate, however, would not receive the added benefits associated with family planning.
4+5 Rural Development and Family Planning	Rural development plus family planning would result in some efficiency-gains in agriculture and—with some decline in family size due to the acceptability of family-planning information—might improve per-capita income. Such interventions would tend to reach only the already-literate adults unless the program were focused toward illiterate adults, or combined with adult-literacy programs. If rural-development innovations decreased reliance on family labor and increased old-age security of families, the result might be greater acceptance of family-planning information.
1+2+3 Nutrition, Public Health, and Education	Better-nourished, healthier children would benefit from better schools, eventually becoming more productive adults. This set of interventions helps children whose poor health and nutrition would have limited their growth and development, and likelihood of participating in school. Nutritional intervention, in the long run, would create dependence on food assistance and should be offered as a short-term intervention

Intervention	Discussion
	only—that is, until long-term benefits can be realized from the higher productivity of educated adults.
1+2+4 Nutrition with Public Health and Rural Development	Increased nutritional intake for the short run, with enhanced rural assistance in the long run, will help food intake. Expanded public-health measures will increase the benefits of food. Higher infant survival probably will result from introduction of public-health measures; this may prevent per-capita income from increasing. On the other hand, increased efficiency of farmers may lead to the increased opportunity of children to attend school instead of working. In the long run, better-educated children will become more efficient farmers and women who may want smaller families. This appears an equitable and efficient combination of interventions.
1+2+5 Nutrition with Public Health and Family Planning	Healthier, better-fed children do better in school. More surviving offspring will lead to bigger families, though increased family-planning interventions may help to encourage limiting births. Eventually, increased literacy and schooling will lead to more productive adults who may desire fewer children.
1+3+4 Nutrition, Education, and Rural Development	This combination will benefit most children whose health permits full use of their nutritional intake. For them, nutritional supplementation probably will lead to greater growth and better school performance. Rural education probably will affect productivity of literate farmers, and lead to enhanced income for that group.
1+3+5 Nutrition, Education, and Family Planning	This combination will benefit most children who are healthy enough to derive full value from their nutrients. This set of interventions would lead to improved growth, development, and school performance for those children. Family planning would be especially acceptable to literate mothers, and to families that do not need to rely on children's economic help.
1+4+5 Nutrition with Rural Development and Family Planning	Improved diet would benefit most those children with adequate health. Rural development and family planning would benefit most literate adults. As before, we see that it is inefficient to improve diet without improving health.

Intervention	Discussion
2+3+4 Public Health with Education and Rural De- velopment	This combination will tend to decrease morbidity; healthier children will be more likely to attend school and perform well. Rural development will enhance agricultural production. For literate and innovative farmers this will be especially beneficial. Eventually, through increased production, diet at home might improve. In the absence of family-planning programs, however, family size may increase with these improved health conditions and, thus, per-capita food availability might not rise. Lack of a nutritional intervention here detracts from an impact on the malnourished poor.
2+3+5 Public Health with Education and Family Planning	Public-health programs and family planning together with improved education will lead to higher school attendance. Family-planning and public-health programs already have been seen to be complementary. Adding investments in education may increase school participation and have beneficial effects on economic productivity. Because of the absence of a nutritional intervention, however, the malnourished would not be helped.
3+4+5 Education with Rural Develop- ment and Family Planning	A combination of educational inputs with rural development and family planning will benefit most those children already able to attend school. Literate adults will tend to benefit from the rural development and family-planning interventions. This tends to benefit those who already have been able to take advantage of schooling.
2+4+5 Public Health with Rural De- velopment and Family Planning	This set of interventions would tend to improve chances of infant survival while working also to limit family size. However, family planning will best help literate mothers who already have less need for the children's work. Rural development programs will help raise economic productivity but will most benefit literate farmers. This rewards those families with education. In the long run, as children's school performance improves with better health, more education will enable them as adults to participate more fully in agricultural innovation.

Intervention	Discussion
1+2+3+4 Nutrition with Public Health, Education, and Rural Development	In the short run, increased nutritional intake together with public health, education, and rural development will help children to be better nourished, healthier, bigger, and better able to perform in school. In the long run, farmers who can acquire literacy will achieve higher productivity. With this set of interventions there is the danger that family size will grow larger because of decreased morbidity and that, although income and food may increase, per-capita income and dietary intake may not.
1+2+3+5 Nutrition with Public Health, Education, and Family Planning	This combination would tend to help the neediest children to achieve better health, growth, and school performance and could balance decreased infant mortality with more acceptance of family planning.
1+2+4+5 Nutrition with Public Health, Rural Development, and Family Planning	This set includes all sectors except additional investments in education. Nutritional improvement plus health would increase the participation and achievement of children who would probably otherwise fail to attend or to perform well. Agricultural assistance and family planning would, in the long run, benefit most literate adults. With larger numbers of children attending school, it might be necessary to increase spending on schools. Nutritional interventions would not be necessary for the long run, as increased productivity would assist eventually in improving family diet.
1+3+4+5 Nutrition with Education, Rural Development, and Family Planning	This includes all sectors except public health. Nutritional intervention therefore would be wasted, since those with diarrheal infection would not be able to use additional nutrients effectively. The additional investment in education would tend to reach children already able to attend school. The rural-development and family-planning information would tend to benefit farmers already innovating, as well as literate mothers.

Intervention	Discussion
2+3+4+5 Public Health, Education, Rural Development, and Family Planning	Since this set does not include nutrition, it prevents immediate assistance to children of the poorest and most malnourished families. These children will be only partly helped by decreased morbidity. The combination of education, rural development, and family planning would appear to be effective in the long run in improving economic productivity and decreasing family size.
1+2+3+4+5 Nutrition, Public Health, Education, Rural Development, and Family Planning	This is the most complete and most ambitious set of interventions. The nutritional intervention should be used only as a short-run benefit for those who need it most. In combination with improved health (and decreased morbidity and infant mortality), children would function better in school. In the long run, educated adults would tend to be more productive and more accepting of family-planning information. In the short run, due to increased child survival, it would be important to focus family-planning programs on those mothers not yet reached because of lack of education. If resources were available, this set of interventions would offer the greatest opportunity for change.

Deciding among Alternatives

To choose among alternative interventions requires agreement about criteria; which criterion will dominate depends on the priorities and values of those with the power to decide. It is much more difficult to predict the consequences of such decisions.

We view criteria for choice among alternatives as being of two kinds: (1) those that would select efficient interventions—that is, those that can achieve agreed-upon goals for the least cost and take advantage of complementarities among programs; or (2) those that would tend to achieve greater equity, being directed particularly toward children and families in greatest need.

Since school success has been shown to depend largely on adequate prior nutritional intake and health, interventions to improve diet and health may give children a better chance to achieve literacy. Thus, if educational programs are accompanied by nutrition and health interventions that benefit children in early childhood, such interventions will improve the effectiveness of educational performance. Children who would benefit most through improved nutrition and health would be just those children who previously would have failed in school.

School participation and achievement also have been found to depend on family affluence and potential needs for children's work. Healthier and more vigorous children could take on both work and school attendance. Children's nutrition and health depend on family affluence. Programs that raise income will in turn improve children's nutrition, health status, and school success.

We do not believe nutritional intervention to be necessary (or advisable) for the long run. A short-term program of nutritional intervention can benefit children of the present generation and increase their long-run opportunities. Long-term intervention of this kind, however, could lead to increased dependence of families on food aid. For the long run, we recommend, rather, measures to increase agricultural production and incomes.

Public-health interventions need to be provided for the long run, and such relatively cheap investments are highly effective. A well that supplies potable water to a community is not costly, nor are latrines. Such services are particularly beneficial since, in the absence of infection, the body's use of nutrients is substantially improved.

Our results show the advantages of immediate institution of public-health interventions with increased nutritional intake (in the short run, by supplementation, family food allotments; and in the long run, by measures to improve productivity). If such programs are undertaken, we would expect children's school performance also to improve, thereby increasing the efficiency of investments in schools.

The literacy and grade-attainment levels of adults are preconditions for accepting innovation in agricultural production and for adopting more positive attitudes with respect to family planning. Literate farmers tend to be more open to rural innovation,* and literate mothers tend to be more accepting of family-planning information.† To increase the investment in either rural development or family planning without increasing the stock of educated and literate

---

* Rural innovation depends also on the quality and quantity of land available.

† Attitudes favorable to family planning depend also on the economic conditions of the family.

adults would be wasteful in the long run, since otherwise acceptance of measures would tend to be limited. Thus, the best approach would be to expand education for children so that the increased benefits of rural development and family-planning interventions would be taking effect as that generation reaches adulthood. For the present generation of adults rural development and family-planning programs either would need to be combined with adult literacy programs or should emphasize outreach to illiterate adults.

In summary, some programs offer interventions that reach children of the poorest groups—those who are generally malnourished and who suffer from diarrheal infection that limits physical growth. These children need, in the short run, and early in life, some form of nutritional intervention combined with improved health conditions. Although the results of our study are specific to the nutritional experiment performed (and we have not studied other forms of supplementation and nutritional change), we do see that increasing protein consumption has a positive effect. We also believe it desirable to increase food intake, but do not believe that calorie supplementation alone will improve children's growth and development.

In addition, by improving health, nutrition, and the quality of the schools, the combined effect upon children will be increased school participation and grade completion. Although we have not specifically studied the quality of the education provided, we have seen that, at existing levels, education and literacy do appear to make a difference in economic opportunity. We believe that if school quality were improved, parental decisions related to children's schooling would reflect the higher quality of the education provided.

In the longer run, for the next generation, it will be necessary to promote the acceptance of lower family size along with acceptance of agricultural innovation. This will be accompanied over time by the greater literacy and grade attainment of the present group of children. To promote acceptance of family planning and rural innovation before the present generation reaches adulthood, it would be advisable to develop programs targeted at illiterate adults.

Because receptivity to family planning depends also on perceiving a reduced need for the children's present work and future help, improvement in the long-run expectations of families about their economic security is called for. By helping farmers achieve greater productivity at the same time that infant mortality is being reduced, we believe that attitudes about desirable family size can be changed.

Here, in summary form, are the strongest predicted policy consequences that stem from our research:

1. Improvements in nutritional intake and improvements in public health should be coupled.
2. Educational investments should be accompanied by improvements in health and nutrition.
3. Rural development is more accepted by literate adults.
4. Family planning is more accepted by literate adults.

Of secondary importance as policy findings, but nevertheless significant as predicted consequences, we also suggest the following:

5. Nutritional improvement should focus on the youngest children.
6. Rural development and family-planning programs should be linked, so that per-capita improvements in income occur as the perceived economic need for children is reduced.
7. Educational quality should be improved to increase school participation which, in the long run, will help to expand innovation and raise productivity.
8. In the short run, until there is greater school participation, rural-development and family-planning programs must be designed and directed especially to the needs of illiterate adults.

We have tried in this book to sort out a few of the important relationships that affect the lives of malnourished children of the rural poor as exemplified by the children in these Guatemalan villages. This was possible because of the existence of the longitudinal nutrition experiment which allowed us to trace changes that came about when malnourished children were offered nutritional supplements. We were also able to evaluate the changes in school participation that resulted from the nutritional intervention. Intergenerational outcomes indicated that schooling affected both the economic productivity of men who farm and the attitudes of women about desirable family size.

This study, and others based on the INCAP experiment, should contribute to microplanning efforts by providing an analytical foundation based on longitudinal data. In the wide variety of countries that need to undertake microplanning to alleviate rural poverty, the basic longitudinal foundations of this study can be supplemented and adjusted by recourse to relatively inexpensive and quick cross-sectional surveys.

We believe that our work also will contribute to macroplanning by providing deeper analytical background and by supplying more reliable parameters, based on micro-analysis, for specifying the behavior of social aggregates. We like to think that our work will lead to further recognition of these complex relationships and to the need for integrated planning. This knowledge, we hope, will lead to greater opportunities for those who otherwise would probably continue to live in poverty.

References

BERG, ALAN, and ROBERT MUSCAT. "Nutrition Program Planning: An Approach." In *Nutrition, National Development, and Planning*, edited by Alan Berg, Nevin Scrimshaw, and David Call. Cambridge, Mass.: MIT Press, 1973.

CHURCHMAN, C. WEST. *The Systems Approach*. New York: Dell Publishing Co., 1979.

EASTERLIN, RICHARD. "The Economics and Sociology of Fertility: A Synthesis." In *Early Industrialization, Shifts in Fertility, and Changes in Family Structure*, edited by C. Tilly. Princeton, N.J.: Princeton University Press, 1977.

GROSSE, ROBERT H., and OSCAR HARKANY. "The Role of Health in Development." *Social Science and Medicine 14C* (1980):165–169.

JOHNSTON, BRUCE. "Food, Health, and Population in Development." *Journal of Economic Literature 15* (September 1977):879–907.

JOHNSTON, BRUCE, and ANTHONY MEYER. "Nutrition, Health, and Population in Strategies for Rural Development." *Economic Development and Cultural Change*, October 1977.

LEIBENSTEIN, HARVEY. "An Interpretation of the Economic Theory of Fertility." *Journal of Economic Literature 12* (1974):457–479.

McEVERS, NORMAN C. "Health and the Assault on Poverty in Low Income Countries." *Social Science and Medicine 14C* (1980):41–57.

MUSHKIN, SELMA. "Educational Outcomes and Nutrition." In *Evaluating the Impact of Nutrition and Health Programs*, edited by R. E. Klein, M. S. Read, H. W. Riecken, J. A. Brown, A. Pradilla, and C. H. Daza. New York: Plenum Press, 1979.

READ, MERRILL S. "Malnutrition, Hunger, and Behavior." *Journal of the American Dietetic Association 63* (October 1973):386–391.

TAYLOR, C. E., and R. D. SINGH, et al. *The Narangwal Population Study: Integrated Health and Family Planning Services*. Punjab, India: Rural Health Research Center, 1975.

WINIKOFF, BEVERLY, and GEORGE BROWN. "Nutrition, Population and Health: Theoretical and Practical Issues." *Social Science and Medicine 14C* (1980):171–176.

INDEX

199

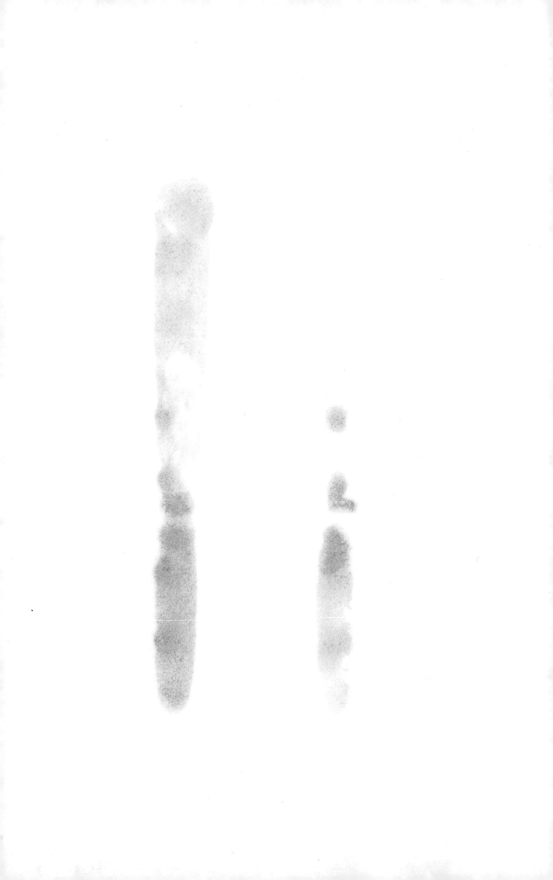

HV
747
,G9
M34

Malnourished child-
ren of the rural
poor

104451

DATE DUE

JUL 2 4 1987		
MAR 3 0 1995		
MAR 2 0 2000		

GAYLORD 234   PRINTED IN U.S.A.

COLLEGE OF MARIN LIBRARY

KENTFIELD, CALIFORNIA

3 2555 00005598 3

CCM

SEP 2 6 1983